Rosemary Gladstar's

Herbs *for the* HOME MEDICINE CHEST

STOREY BOOKS

*The mission of Storey Communications is to serve our customers
by publishing practical information that encourages
personal independence in harmony with the environment.*

This publication is intended to provide educational information for the
reader on the covered subject. It is not intended to take the place of
personalized medical counseling, diagnosis, and treatment from a trained
health professional.

Edited by Deborah Balmuth and Robin Catalano
Cover design by Carol Jessop, Black Trout Design, and Meredith Maker
Back cover photograph by A. Blake Gardner
Cover and interior illustrations by Laura Tedeschi
Text design by Carol Jessop, Black Trout Design
Text production by Susan B. Bernier
Indexed by Nan Badgett, Word•a•bil•i•ty

Copyright © 1999 by Rosemary Gladstar

Sections of this book previously appeared in the author's self-published booklet
titled *Herbal Medicinal Preparations* (1989).

All rights reserved. No part of this book may be reproduced without written
permission from the publisher, except by a reviewer who may quote brief passages or reproduce illustrations in a review with appropriate credits; nor may
any part of this book be reproduced, stored in a retrieval system, or transmit-
ted in any form or by any means — electronic, mechanical, photocopying, record-
ing, or other — without written permission from the publisher.

The information in this book is true and complete to the best of our knowledge. All recommendations are made without guarantee on the part of the author
or Storey Books. The author and publisher disclaim any liability in connection
with the use of this information. For additional information please contact Storey
Books, Schoolhouse Road, Pownal, Vermont 05261.

Storey Books are available for special premium and promotional uses and
for customized editions. For further information, please call the Custom Publishing Department at 1-800-793-9396.

Printed in Canada by Webcom Limited
10 9 8 7 6 5 4 3

Library of Congress Cataloging-in-Publication Data

Gladstar, Rosemary.
   [Herbs for the home medicine chest]
   Rosemary Gladstar's herbs for the home medicine chest / Rosemary Gladstar.
     p.   cm.
   Includes bibliographical references and index.
   ISBN 1-58017-156-7 (pbk. : alk. paper)
   1. Herbs — Therapeutic use.   I. Title.
RM666.H33G534   1999
615'.321—dc21   99-19955
                                                    CIP

Dedication

There is a circle, green hands enfolded, lives entwined, of fellow herbalists. I've held each of their hands and laughed and prayed with them, these old friends who influenced my earliest teachings. Their thoughts are embedded in my heart and flow into the words of this book.

It has been almost two decades since we first met at the earliest herb gatherings in Sonoma County. We offered some of our original herb classes and went on some of our earliest herb walks together. At a time when herbalism wasn't popular or faddish, we "followed our bliss," our green passion. Now practically elders, ever more empassioned by the green world, we face a new millennium, wondering not what the world has in store for herbalism but what the herbs have in store for us.

One always runs the risk of forgetting someone very important as the night lights fade and the years draw on, but for this moment, I'm remembering these faces from 20 years ago: Svevo Brooks, Nan Koehler, Rob Menzies, Jeannie Rose, Ed Smith, Christopher Hobbs, Michael Tierra, Sara Katz, Gabrielle Howearth, Cascade Anderson Geller, James Green, Kathi Keville, Jesse Longacre, Ryan Drum, Mindy Green, Selena Heron, Steven Foster, Mark Blumenthal, Warren Raysor, Jeannine Parvati Baker, Nam Singh, David Winston, and Michael Moore.

May the circle ever grow and the weeds be plentiful.

Acknowledgments

I am sincerely indebted and grateful to the endless support and hard work of my editors Robin Catalano and Deborah Balmuth. Their patience and caring sustained me through endless deadlines amidst a schedule that was nothing less than chaotic. Due to their understanding, the help of the nervine herbs, and the view out my office window, I'm alive and well at the end of this writing odyssey. I'd also like to thank fellow herbalists Amy Goodman and Cheryl Hartt for their help with Making Your Own First-Aid Kit.

CONTENTS

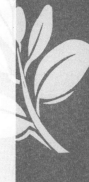

chapter one

Understanding Herbs

I was at a large conference recently participating in a panel of "experts" on herbal medicine. Each person on the panel had been involved in herbal studies for more than two decades and was quite well known, not to mention knowledgeable about the subject. It was a long workshop, with each presenter discussing a different aspect of herbal medicine. I think we all felt fairly good about the perspectives we were sharing and the overviews we had given, but when it came time for questions and answers, the very first question came from a woman sitting in the front row who had been listening intently the entire time. She stated quite simply, "I came here hoping to gain some clarity about how to use herbs for myself and my family and I'm more confused than ever." This book is written for that woman.

The Healing Powers of Plants

For ages, long before we had computers, technology, libraries, or even herb books, people knew and understood the healing power of herbs. I am convinced that this knowing came from an intrinsic sense of the plant. It was not simply a trial-and-error process by which people learned about the plant spirit and medicine, as we often postulate. Plants have an innate way of communicating with people. And though I believe that almost anybody can learn to listen to the plants, there are certain people who lend an ear more readily to the voices of the plants. These people are generally termed keepers of the green, green witches, herbalists, or healers.

Ancient Herbalism

In traditional cultures the herb gatherers were trained to ask permission from the plant itself before harvesting it for medicine. This was considered not only essential for retaining the healing power of the plant, but also respectful, a simple courtesy. When trying to determine a remedy or an appropriate treatment, you should consider asking the plant directly, not in place of adequate research and study, but in addition to it. Try "consulting" with the plants as part of the

MAYAN PRAYER FOR PICKING PLANTS?

In the name of God the Father, God the Son, and God the Holy Spirit, I am the one searching for the plants to heal the people. I give thanks to the spirit of this plant, and I have faith with all my heart that this plant will heal the sickness of [person's name].

process. The plants are here to help us; asking for their help is one step in understanding them.

When I'm harvesting plants for medicine, I first ask the plant's permission to use its healing power. And sometimes when I'm trying to find an appropriate remedy or combination of herbs, I ask the plants directly and I get a feeling about which plant is right. This isn't a special gift, it's a gift many people have, but most forget how to use it. As you become more familiar working with plants and using herbal remedies, this skill begins to ripen and mature and becomes a guiding light in your of understanding plant medicine. Again, it doesn't replace book learning, but augments it.

When to Use Herbs

With all of the possibilities of health care offered today, making a wise choice can be challenging. What is the most responsible thing to do? Each situation is different, of course. In one instance antibiotics and a hospital visit may be a wise choice; in another situation herbal remedies and home treatments may be the most responsible approach to take. So how does one decide?

Home Health Care with Herbs

Basically, if your grandmother would have treated the problem at home, you probably can too. This is a sweeping statement, I know, and there are many exceptions to it. Though it can be, and is, effectively used for complex health situations, even life-threatening situations at times, herbalism is at its best as a home health care system.

Most illnesses and imbalances respond to nourishment, rest, and gentle natural treatments. If your body does not respond in an appropriate manner or does not respond quickly enough for the situation, then consider consulting a medical practitioner, ideally one who is interested in and knowledgeable about holistic treatments. Unless your health care practitioner is educated about herbs, he or she will not be able to give you good advice on the use of herbs.

Complementing Allopathic Health Care

Herbalism and allopathic medicine often seem at odds with one another. But they are, in fact, complementary and can work compatibly, enhancing the possibilities for well-being. Though some of the strongest herbs should not be used with allopathic drugs, most herbs do not interfere with the actions of chemical drugs and can be used to augment allopathic treatments.

While allopathic drugs actively kill bacteria and viruses, herbal medicines build and restore the system. Allopathic medication generally has a specific agenda; herbs, through a complex biochemical process, take the whole person into consideration and replenish from a cellular level. When taken correctly, herbs do not upset the body's innate sense of harmony, so there are few or no side effects. Using herbal therapies with chemical drugs often helps eliminate or lessen the side effects of drug therapies.

Using Herbal Medicine

Each situation requiring medical attention is different. But here are some guidelines for recognizing when herbal treatments can be better than allopathic treatments:

As preventive medicine. Herbs are inimitable for building and strengthening the body's natural immunity and defense mechanisms. They nourish the deep inner ecology of our systems on a cellular level. Herbs are also powerful adaptogens, increasing the body's ability to adapt to the ever-changing environment and increased stresses of life. Our bodies are familiar with herbs, recognize them, and efficiently utilize them.

Most nonemergency medical situations. Everyday problems such as bruises, swellings, sprains, cuts, wounds, colds, fevers, and burns respond well to herbalism. Herbs can also be an effective first-aid treatment for emergency situations when medical help is unavailable or on its way.

As therapeutic agents. If one chooses to undergo more radical forms of treatment for treating serious illnesses such as cancer, AIDS, and other autoimmune disorders, herbs serve as excellent secondary therapeutic agents, supporting and replenishing the life energy. Herbs and allopathic medicine work compatibly in these critical situations and can be used to complement and enhance the effects of one another.

Getting Perspective on the Safety of Using Herbs

Herbs are among the safest medications available on earth. This does not mean that there are not toxic plants or herbal remedies that can cause side effects or harmful reactions in the body. In fact, some of the deadliest substances on earth are found in plants such as *Amanita phalloides,* or death cap mushroom. But this system of healing has been practiced for several thousand years. The herbs we use today have been used for centuries by people around the world.

What About Adverse Reactions?

Herbs that have toxic side effects have been noted and well documented; most of these herbs, wisely, are not available for sale in this country. Occasionally, an herb will stimulate an idiosyncratic reaction in an individual. This doesn't make the herb toxic, just a poor choice for that particular individual. Strawberries, a perfectly delicious fruit, are sweet nectar to some and a noxious substance to others.

There are many reports surfacing these days about the toxicity of herbs. Even perfectly benign substances such as chamomile and peppermint are finding themselves on the "black list." I think the reason for this is not that more people are using herbs, as is often suggested, but that people are using herbs in ways that allow greater and more concentrated dosages. In the past, herbs were most often taken as teas and syrups, in baths and salves, and in tinctures and extracts. But herbal capsules, which allow people to swallow as many as they wish, and standardized preparations, which are far beyond the normal concentrations found in nature, have not been available until recently.

Any herb, even the safest and most researched of herbs, can affect different people differently. Though it is a rare occurrence, whenever such a reaction is reported it makes national headlines and creates a certain alarm among plant users. Were drug reactions reported with the same fervor, we'd have a national headline on aspirin every day. However rare these reactions to herbs may be, it is always wise to practice caution when using an herb for the first time, especially when using it on your children.

With not centuries but millennia of experience behind the use of medicinal herbs, you can be assured of their safety. Follow the appropriate dosages outlined in this book (see page 14 for a general dosage chart), use only those herbs that have a record of safety, and respond quickly by discontinuing an herb if you suspect it is causing an idiosyncratic response.

THE SAFETY OF MEDICINAL HERBS

In 1997 approximately 100,000 people in the United States died from adverse reactions to legal prescription drugs. Between 5,000 and 10,000 deaths due to illicit drugs were reported. If there were any deaths due to the use of medicinal herbs, they were not reported. The American Association of Poison Control Centers (AAPCC) receives so few toxicity reports due to medicinal herb usage that there is no special category assigned to them. The AAPCC reports that herbs are not a major public health hazard, while houseplants and mushrooms account for a great number of poisonings each year, as do prescription and over-the-counter drugs.

chapter two

The Art
of Making
Herbal Remedies

It took some years to develop these recipes and formulas, and it is with pleasure that I pass them along to you. When I first began working with herbs in the late 1960s, what little explanation there was on how to prepare herbs was difficult to find. Often the steps were complicated and sometimes the herbs mentioned were not even available. Through a wonderful creative process of trial and error, learning from the old masters and their books, and sharing with and learning from my friends, the instructions for these preparations began to take shape. Included in this chapter is the information I wish I had when I first began to study herbs so many years ago.

Buying and Storing Herbs

It is important when using herbs that you insist on high-quality organically grown herbs. Though these herbs may cost a few cents more, they are far better for our medicines and, ultimately, our planet. Have at least two ounces of the herbs you plan to use on hand at all times. And don't use herbs that are endangered or at risk, whether from this country or elsewhere; it is critical when using herbs today that each person takes responsibility for where the herbs are coming from and who is growing and harvesting them. To learn more about endangered herbs, contact United Plant Savers (see Resources).

Purchasing Herbs

How do you tell if a dried herb is of good quality? It should look, taste, and smell almost exactly as it does when fresh, and it should be effective. Dried herbs should still have vibrant color, and they should smell strongly, though not necessarily "good." Herbs should have a distinctive, fresh flavor. Do not judge them on taste by expecting them to taste "good"; judge taste on potency rather than flavor. Finally, if the herbs you are using are not working as you well as would expect them to, inspect the quality of the herb first.

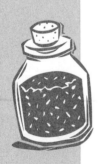

I have traveled in various parts of the world, and I am astounded by the differences in the quality of the herbs. Originally, the quality of herbs in the United States was very poor, but in the last 25 years there has been such an emphasis placed on using high-quality herbs that we now lead the world in quality standards.

We are hoping we will have the same influence worldwide on preservation as we have had on quality. If we wish to preserve this system of healing for our children as it has been passed down to us from our ancestors, preservation of medicinal plant species becomes imperative. You are supporting not only your own health but the health of the planet when you buy organically.

Growing Your Own Medicinal Herb Garden

The best way to assure you're getting quality herbs is to grow your own. Many of the plants that you use for medicine can be grown as part of your vegetable and flower garden. Incorporate them into your landscape and use them as they grow and thrive. Though many have specific habitats and limited range, which is one reason why they are threatened, we are finding that many of them are far more adaptable than was previously thought. For an excellent book on the subject, read *Medicinal Herbs in the Garden, Field, and Marketplace* by Tim Blakley and Lee Sturdivant. See page 55 for a list of plants that are useful in home health care and are under stress in their natural habitats due to overharvesting or habitat destruction.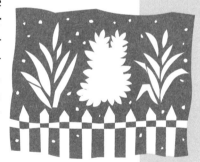

How to Store Herbs

Herbs retain their properties best if stored in airtight glass jars, away from direct light, in a cool storage area. For convenience, you can store them in many other containers — boxes, tins, plastic bags — but most conscientious herbalists find those durable glass bottles the best for storage.

Each herb has its own "shelf life," and following a set rule could mean you would throw out perfectly fine peppermint while using poor-quality chickweed. Use the "quality-control test" on page 8 to determine if your herbs have retained their quality.

The Kitchen "Lab"

A kitchen, with all of its marvelous tools, will supply you with most of the utensils you need for preparing herbal products. One of the few rules that most herbalists agree on is never to use aluminum pots and pans for preparing herbs. In spite of its popularity, aluminum is a proven toxic substance that is easily released by heat into our food. Use glass, stainless steel, ceramic, cast iron, or enamel cooking equipment.

Some items I've found especially useful are:

- Cheesecloth or fine muslin for straining herbs
- A large, double-meshed stainless steel strainer
- Stainless steel pots with tight-fitting lids
- A grater reserved for grating beeswax
- Canning jars for storing herbs and making tinctures
- Measuring cups (though, heaven forbid, I hardly use them)
- A coffee grinder for grinding herbs (Don't use your herb grinder for coffee. You'll forever have the flavor of herbs in your coffee and the scent of coffee in your herbs.)

How to Determine Measurements

While many people are converting to the metric system, I've reverted to the Simpler's method of measuring. Many herbalists choose to use this system because it is extremely simple and very versatile. Throughout this book you'll see measurements referred to as "parts": 3 parts chamomile,

SCIENCE AND HERBAL HEALING

Long before the term *herbalist* was coined, people who worked closely with the earth, plants, and the seasons were called simplers. Not a derogatory term at all, a simpler was observant and relied on intuition and an inner knowing. Over the centuries, science developed weights and measures and clinical studies to comprehend, measure, and explain this art of healing. A tablespoon or two of this clinical knowledge is appropriate to the study of herbs, and adds a touch of professionalism to the art. More than that, I'm afraid, could be toxic to the creative unfolding of herbal healing.

1 part lemon balm, 2 parts oats. The use of the word "part" allows the measurement to be determined in relation to the other ingredients. A part is a unit of measurement that can be interpreted to mean cups, ounces, pounds, tablespoons, or teaspoons — as long as you use that unit consistently throughout the recipe. If you were using tablespoons in the recipe above, you would include 3 tablespoons of chamomile, 1 tablespoon of lemon balm, and 2 tablespoons of oats.

Herbal Teas

Herbal teas remain my favorite way of using herbs medicinally. The mere act of making tea and drinking it involves you in the healing process and, I suspect, awakens an innate sense of healing in you. Though medicinal teas are generally not as potent or as active as tinctures and other concentrated herbal remedies, they are the most effective medicines for chronic, long-term imbalances. And all you really need is a quart jar with a tight-fitting lid, the selected herbs, and water that has reached the boiling point.

Herbal teas can be drunk hot, at room temperature, or iced. They can be made into ice cubes with fresh fruit and flowers and used to flavor festive holiday punches. They're delicious blended with fruit juice and frozen as pops for children.

Once brewed, an herbal tea should be stored in the refrigerator. Left at room temperature for several hours, it will go "flat," get tiny bubbles in it, and begin to sour. Stored in the refrigerator, an herbal tea is good for three to four days.

I seldom direct people to make medicinal teas by the cupful. It is impractical and time consuming. Instead, make a quart of tea each morning or in the evening after work. Use four to six tablespoons of herb per quart of water. The herb-to-water ratio varies, depending on the quality of herbs used, whether the herb is fresh or dried (use twice as much fresh herb in a recipe), and how strong you wish the finished tea to be. There are two basic methods for making tea, and two variations I've included just for fun.

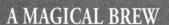

A MAGICAL BREW

Many years ago when I was a carefree young woman, I wished for a partner. I made a list of qualities I thought were important. Then I brewed a magical goblet of tea. I stirred in the perfect flowers picked from my garden, and an amethyst crystal for the heart. I placed that goblet filled with wishes on my porch railing, in the path of the radiant August moonlight. The next morning, upon waking, I drank every drop of that divinely delicious tea. Did I meet my prince? Well, of course, or I'd not be telling the tale. And I did learn how powerful these teas really are, so be careful what you wish for.

FRESH OR DRIED HERBS?

There is nothing quite as good as the taste of fresh picked herbs. However many herbs are not available fresh year-round, and some of our favorite herbs are not grown in this country but are dried and imported. When fresh herbs are unavailable, high-quality dried herbs will do just fine. Fresh herb blends must be used immediately, of course, while dried mixtures can be stored for several months or longer.

Infusions

Infusions are made from the more delicate parts of the plant, including the leaves, flowers, and aromatic parts. Place the herb in a quart jar, or any container with a tight-fitting lid, and pour boiling water over it. Cover; let steep for 30 to 45 minutes. A longer steeping time will make a stronger tea.

Decoctions

Decoctions are made from the more tenacious parts of the plant, such as the roots and bark. It's a little harder to extract the constituents from these parts, so a slow simmer (or an overnight infusion) is often required. Place herbs in a small saucepan and cover with cold water. Heat slowly and simmer, with the lid on, for 20 to 45 minutes. Again, the longer you simmer the herbs, the stronger the tea will be.

Solar and Lunar Infusions

Have you ever considered using the light of the moon or the sun for extracting the healing properties of the herbs? It's one of my favorite methods for making herbal tea. Sometimes after I've prepared a tea on my kitchen stove, I'll place it in the moonlight or sunlight to pick up some of the rays of these giant luminaries. We are children of the sky as well as the earth; using the energies of the stars and moon and sun in our healing work adds a special touch.

Solar tea is made by placing the herbs and water in a glass jar with a tight-fitting lid. Place directly in the hot sunlight for several hours.

Lunar tea is made by placing the herbs and water in an open container (unless there are lots of night flying bugs around!) and positioning it directly in the path of the moonlight. Lunar tea is subtle and magical; it is whispered that fairies love to drink it.

Dosage Chart for Adults

Chronic Problems include long-term imbalances such as hay fever, arthritis, and long-standing bronchial problems. Chronic problems can, however, flare up with acute symptoms. Follow these guidelines for treating chronic problems.

TEA	EXTRACTS/ TINCTURES*	CAPSULES/ TABLETS
3–4 cups daily for several weeks	½–1 teaspoon 3 times daily	2 capsules 3 times daily

Acute Problems are sudden, reaching a crisis and needing quick attention. Examples of acute problems include toothaches, wounds, bleeding, and sudden onset of cold or flu. Follow these guidelines for treating acute problems.

TEA	EXTRACTS/ TINCTURES*	CAPSULES/ TABLETS
¼–½ cup served throughout the day, up to 3–4 cups	¼–½ teaspoon every 30–60 minutes until symptoms subside	1 capsule every hour until symptoms subside

*includes syrups and elixirs

Syrups

Syrups are the yummiest of all herbal preparations. Because they are sweet, children often prefer their medicine in this form. They are delicious, concentrated extracts of the herbs cooked into a sweet medicine with the addition of honey and/or fruit juice. Vegetable glycerin may be substituted for honey; it is an excellent medium for the herbs and is very nutritious for children.

This is my favorite method for making syrup:

Step 1. Use two ounces of herb mixture to one quart of water. Over low heat, simmer the liquid down to one pint. This will give you a very concentrated, thick tea.

Step 2. Strain the herbs from the liquid. Compost the herbs and pour the liquid back into the pot.

Step 3. To each pint of liquid, add one cup of honey (or other sweetener such as maple syrup, vegetable glycerin, or brown sugar). Most recipes call for two cups of sweetener (a 1:1 ratio of sweetener to liquid). I find it far too sweet for my taste, but the added sugar helped preserve the syrup in the days when refrigeration wasn't common.

Step 4. Warm the honey and liquid together only enough to mix well. Most recipes instruct you to cook for 20 to 30 minutes longer over high heat to thicken further. It does certainly make thicker syrup, but I'd rather not cook the living enzymes out of the honey.

Step 5. When finished heating, you may add a fruit concentrate to flavor, or a couple of drops of essential oil such as peppermint or spearmint, or a small amount of brandy to help preserve the syrup and to aid as a relaxant in cough formulas.

Step 6. Remove from the heat and bottle for use. Syrups will last for several weeks, even months, if refrigerated.

Herbal Candy

Far more delightful than taking herbs in tinctures or pill form are these delicious medicinal "candies." You can mix just about any herbal formula this way. By carefully measuring the amount of herbs and the number of balls you make, you can calculate fairly accurately an appropriate daily dose.

To make herbal candy:

1. Grind raisins, dates, apricots, and walnuts in a food processor or grinder. Alternatively, you can mix nut butter (such as peanut, almond, or cashew) with honey in equal portions. *Note:* If you're concerned about the use of honey (due to reports of botulism), then use maple syrup, rice syrup, or maple cream.
2. Stir in shredded coconut and carob powder.
3. Mix in the herb powders well.
4. Roll mixture into balls. Roll again in powdered carob or coconut. Store in refrigerator.

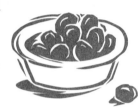

Medicinal Oils

Herbal oils are simple to make, and may be used as a base for salves and ointments. By using different combinations of herbs and oils, you can make either strong medicinal oils or sweet-scented massage and bath oils. Though any good-quality vegetable oil may be used, the oil of choice for medicine is olive; there simply is no finer oil for this purpose.

If your herbal oil grows mold, there is either too much water content in the herb or moisture in the jar. Use dry herbs or wilt the herbs before using. Be *absolutely* certain the container is completely dry. Check the lid for moisture; it is often the culprit.

Making Solar-infused Oils

Place herbs and oil in a glass jar; cover tightly. Place the jar in a warm, sunny spot. Let the mixture infuse for two weeks, after which you may strain the oil, add a fresh batch of herbs, and infuse for two more weeks. This will give you a very potent medicinal oil.

Strain well. Use cheesecloth or a muslin cloth to strain. When the oil has been poured off, put the herbs into a separate container and squeeze the remaining oil out thoroughly.

HOW MUCH IS A DROP?

Have you ever been frustrated when a recipe provides one type of measurement only? Here are some basic conversions to keep in mind:

Teaspoons	Droppers Full	Milliliters
¼	1 (35 drops)	1
½	2.5 (88 drops)	2.5
1	5 (175 drops)	5

(Who was it that counted those drops? I'd like to thank her!)

Using the Double Boiler Method

Although it doesn't provide the benefits of the sun, this is a quick and simple method that makes beautiful oil.

Place herbs and oil in a double boiler and bring to a low simmer. Slowly heat for 30 to 60 minutes, checking frequently to be sure the oil is not overheating. The lower the heat, the longer the infusion, the better the oil.

Strain herbal mixture thoroughly. Line a large stainless steel strainer with cheesecloth or muslin. Pour the mixture through. Reserve the oil. Store your finished herbal oil in a cool, dark area. It does not have to be refrigerated, but it will quickly deteriorate in heat. Stored properly, herbal oils will last for several months, sometimes years.

Salves and Ointments

Once you've made herbal oil, you're a step away from a salve. Salves and ointments (basically different terms for the same product) are made of beeswax, herbs, and vegetable (or animal) oils. The oil is used as a solvent for the medicinal properties of the herb and provides a healing, emollient base. The beeswax also adds a soothing, protective quality and provides the firmness necessary to form the salve.

To make a salve:

Step 1. Prepare medicinal oil following instructions above. Strain.

Step 2. To each cup of herbal oil, add ¼ cup beeswax. Heat until the beeswax is completely melted. To check for firmness, place one tablespoon of the mixture in the freezer for just a minute or two. If it's too soft, add more beeswax; if too hard, add more oil.

Step 3. Remove from heat immediately and pour into small glass jars or tins. Store any extra salve in a cool, dark place. Stored properly, salves will last for months, even years. Some people recommend adding natural preservatives to the mixture, such as vitamin E or tincture of benzoin, but I've never found it necessary or any more effective.

Tinctures

Tinctures are concentrated extracts of herbs. They are taken by simply diluting a dropperful or two of the tincture in warm water or juice. Most tinctures are made with alcohol as the primary solvent or extractant. Though the amount of alcohol is very small, many people choose not to use alcohol-based tinctures, especially for children, for a variety of sound reasons. Effective tinctures can be made with vegetable glycerin or apple cider vinegar as the solvent. Though they may not be as strong as alcohol-based preparations, they do work and are preferred for children and people who are alcohol sensitive. Because of its sweet nature, glycerin-based tinctures taste far better than those made with alcohol and they have a long shelf life.

Some of the alcohol in tinctures can be removed by placing the tincture in boiling water for one to two minutes. This method is only effective

HERBAL LINIMENTS?

An herbal liniment is made in *exactly* the same way as a tincture; however, a liniment, which uses rubbing alcohol or witch hazel as its solvent, is for *external* purposes. Liniments are either made for disinfectant purposes or to soothe sore, inflamed muscles.

Follow the directions below to make your liniment. Be sure to label the bottle FOR EXTERNAL USE ONLY to avoid accidents.

for removing about 50 percent of the alcohol; there will always remain some residual alcohol.

Making Herbal Tinctures

There are several methods used to make tinctures. The traditional or Simpler's method is the method I prefer. It is an extremely simple system that produces beautiful tinctures every time. All that is required to make a tincture in the traditional method is the herbs, the menstruum, and a jar with a tight-fitting lid.

Step 1. Chop your herbs finely. I recommend using fresh herbs whenever possible. High-quality dried herbs will work well also, but one of the advantages of tincturing is the ability to preserve the fresh attributes of the plant. Place the herbs in a clean, dry jar.

Step 2. Pour the menstruum over the herbs. If using vegetable glycerin, dilute it with an equal amount of water before pouring over the herbs. If using vinegar as the menstruum, warm the vinegar first to facilitate the release of herbal constituents. If choosing alcohol as your solvent, select one that is 80 to 100 proof (40 percent to 50 percent alcohol), such as vodka, gin, or brandy. *Completely cover* the herbs with the menstruum and then add an additional two to three inches more of liquid. The herbs need to be completely submersed. Cover with a tight-fitting lid.

Step 3. Place the jars in a warm place and let the herbs and liquid soak (macerate) for four to six weeks — the longer, the better. Place the bottles in a place where they will demand daily attention, such as on a kitchen sill or even in the bathroom.

Step 4. I encourage the daily shaking of the bottles of tinctures during the maceration period. This not only prevents the herbs from packing down on the bottom of the jar, but is also an invitation for some of the old magic to come back into medicine making. During the shaking process, you can sing to your tincture jars, stir them in the moonlight or the sunlight, wave feathers over them — whatever your imagination inspires.

Herbal Pills

Herbal pills are simple and practical to make. You can formulate your own blends and make them taste good enough so that even children will eat them. Formulate them with herbs for the throat to make a tasty sore throat remedy to suck on.

To make herbal pills:

Step 1. Place powdered herbs in a bowl and moisten with enough water and honey (or pure Vermont maple syrup) to make a sticky paste.

Step 2. Add a tiny drop of essential oil such as peppermint or wintergreen oil and mix well.

Step 3. Thicken with carob powder. Add enough carob to form a smooth paste. Knead until smooth, like the texture of bread dough.

Step 4. Roll into small balls the size of pills. You can roll again in carob powder for a finished look.

Step 5. Place on a cookie sheet and dry in a very low oven (even the pilot light will work) or sun dry for a day. These pills, once dried, will store indefinitely. I often store mine, undried and unrolled, in the refrigerator in a glass jar with a tight-fitting lid. I roll them as I need them (very unprofessional but it saves time and is just as effective).

Herbal Baths

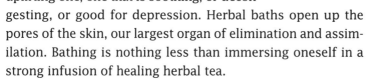

Several prominent healers administer most of their herbal formulas via the bath. Depending on the herbs or herbal formulas you choose and the temperature of the water, you can create either a relaxing bath or a stimulating, uplifting one, one that is soothing, or decongesting, or good for depression. Herbal baths open up the pores of the skin, our largest organ of elimination and assimilation. Bathing is nothing less than immersing oneself in a strong infusion of healing herbal tea.

The water should be warm or hot for a relaxing bath, cool to cold for a stimulating bath, and tepid for a neutral bath. Place the herbs in a large handkerchief, clean nylon stocking, or strainer, and tie it on the nozzle of the tub. Allow the hot water to flow through the herb bag vigorously until about half the tub is filled. Adjust water temperature as desired and continue filling the tub.

Herbal baths may also be administered solely to the feet or hands. All of the nerve endings in the entire body pass through the feet and hands, making them a map of our inner being. Use an appropriate size container.

JULIETTE'S "MIRACLE" BATH

Juliette de Bairacli Levy has had a profound influence on American herbalism.

One time, after an extremely stressful flight from her home in the Azores to visit me in Vermont, Juliette broke out in a terrible bout of shingles. It was the worst case I had ever seen and I was frightened for her life. What great remedy did she use to cure this terrible affliction? Baths of oatmeal sprinkled with lavender oil, and cabbage leaf poultices applied over her entire body.

Gathering the Ingredients

It is wise to assemble all the ingredients and utensils you need ahead of time. There have been times when I haven't followed this little bit of advice, and in the middle of a project found I was out of a necessary ingredient. This can be either a big or little inconvenience, but it's always annoying.

As with any recipe, you can substitute ingredients and experiment with the formulas to create a more personalized product, but be sure you understand what the particular ingredient in the formula is "doing" so that you can substitute one product with another that has similar properties; otherwise the product may not turned out as hoped for. Ask yourself the basic questions: Is this ingredient an emulsifier? Does it help thicken the product? Does it add moisture?

In these recipes there is always lots of room for creativity. I am one of those people who gets frustrated with exact proportions. Coffee cups are most often my measuring cups and spoons from my silverware drawer serve as measuring spoons. When adding essential oils I lose count some where after the fourth or fifth drop and proceed forward by scent and common sense alone. Nothing is exact in my world, and, needless to say, things don't always turn out exactly the same. But I've learned to follow my intuition, and generally it leads me in its own creative process. Using my common sense rather than exact measurements has often produced exquisite results.

WHAT MAKES A GOOD HERBALIST?

My idea of a good herbalist isn't someone who knows the uses of forty different herbs, but someone who knows how to use one herb in forty different ways.

— *Svevo Brooks*

chapter three

The Home Herbal Pantry

Though it's always a challenging task to decide which of the many wonderful herbs to include in listings such as this, I've limited my discussion to those herbs that have the greatest safety record and are commonly used for household situations. Most of these herbs can be used successfully over a long period of time for a variety of purposes. Warnings are given when appropriate. For a more complete listing of beneficial herbs or for further information on the herbs that I have included, consult any one of the encyclopedic herbal compendiums available today.

Reading will fill your head with the wonderful facts and stories about each plant, but herbalism is more than "head" learning. Plants teach by interacting with us, so the best possible way to learn about each herb is to experience it. After you've read about it, if it seems like an herb that is appropriate for your situation, try it. The taste, the smell, the effect of the herb on your being is the best laboratory you have for determining its effectiveness.

When teaching my students how to use herbs, I insist they try each one as a tea. In this way, they learn about its flavor and effects. Next, I ask them to research the herb in several good reference books. This information augments one's direct experience with the herbs.

Listen to the wisdom of your body, the feeling of the herbs as you're using them, and the book knowledge you gain as you read about them.

DO YOUR RESEARCH

I've always felt it a requisite when studying herbs to reference *each* herb you're planning to use in at least *three* different herb books. Because herbs are so multifaceted, no one book will give you a complete picture of what it is or what it can do. But reading about it in several books will give you a broader understanding of the depths and possibilities of each herb you are working with.

Astragalus *(Astragalus membranaceous)*

Parts used: roots

Benefits: Adaptogenic, tonifiying, often called the young person's ginseng, astragalus builds the deep immune system and helps rebuild the bone marrow reserve that regenerates the body's protective shield. It is particularly beneficial for strengthening the spleen and lungs. It is a superior tonic herb and is used in the treatment of chronic imbalances. It is also useful for regulating metabolism of dietary sugars, and thus is helpful for people with diabetes.

Suggested uses: Astragalus is best used in tea for long-term illness, low energy, and to support and build deep immune strength. Place a whole root or two in a pot of soup and simmer several hours. Astragalus can also be served in capsules. It's quite tasty and can be chewed like licorice sticks.

Burdock *(Arctium lappa)*

Parts used: primarily roots and seeds, but leaves can be used externally

Benefits: This tenacious wild plant is a bane to farmers and a blessing to herbalists. It is simply the best herb for the skin and can be used internally and externally for eczema, psoriasis, acne, and other skin-related imbalances. It is a specific for the liver, and because of its pleasant flavor is often formulated with other less tasty "liver herbs."

Suggested uses: Burdock makes a fine-tasting tea and can be adapted for teenagers with problem skin by serving it with juice or other herb teas. It is also used as a wash for itchy, irritated skin. Decoct the root and serve with meals as a digestive aid. The fresh root, grated and steamed and served with a sprinkle of toasted sesame seed oil, is delicious. The seeds are often used in ointments for the skin.

Calendula *(Calendula officinalis)*

Parts used: flowers

Benefits: Known to most people as marigold, this sunny little flower brightens most gardens. It is a powerful vulnerary, healing the body by promoting cell repair, and acts as an antiseptic, keeping infection from occurring in injuries. Calendula is most often used externally for bruises, burns, sores, and skin ulcers. It is also used internally for fevers and for gastrointestinal problems such as ulcers, cramps, indigestion, and diarrhea. And, of course, you see it used in many cosmetics for its skin-soothing effects.

Suggested uses: Marigold is most often used in salves for burns and irritated skin, but it is effective as an infusion for skin problems, fevers, and gastrointestinal upsets. It is oftentimes brewed triple strength and used as a hair rinse.

Cayenne pepper *(Capsicum annuum and related species)*

Parts used: fruits

Benefits: There's a cult growing around the use of cayenne, and it's deserving of all this attention. It serves as a catalyst to the system, stimulating the body's natural defense system. It has antiseptic properties and is an excellent warming circulatory herb. It is one of the best heart tonics, increasing the pulse and toning the heart muscle. Cayenne is a natural coagulant that stops bleeding and, finally, it is an excellent carminative, stimulating the digestive process and helping with congestion and constipation.

Suggested uses: Cayenne can be used sparingly in many formulas (teas, capsules, tinctures, and food preparations) as a catalyst or action herb. The burning feeling it creates is superficial and not harmful.

Caution: Cayenne, though perfectly safe, is hot! Even a pinch of cayenne in a tincture formula can overwhelm, and a grain or more in an herbal pill can send you to the ceiling.

Chamomile (Anthemis nobilis and related species)

Parts used: primarily flowers, but leaves are useful

Benefits: This little plant is a healing wonder. It has rich amounts of essential oil in its flower tops that acts as a powerful anti-inflammatory agent. The flowers make a soothing tea that is good for the nervous system. It is a general digestive aid and is one of the best herbs for colicky babies.

Suggested uses: The tea sweetened with honey can be served throughout the day to calm stress and nervousness. A few drops of chamomile tincture will aid digestion; give before feeding time. Chamomile makes an excellent massage oil for stress and anxiety. Add a few drops of essential oil of chamomile to the massage oil for sore, achy muscles. Chamomile is frequently added to bathwater for a wonderfully relaxing and soothing wash.

Chaste tree (Vitex agnus-castus)

Parts used: berries

Benefits: Chaste tree is a shrub native to the Mediterranean region that has been employed by Europeans since ancient times. It is one of the most important herbs for feeding and nourishing the reproductive organs of men and women and is especially helpful in restoring vitality and general tone to the female system. Vitex is the herb of choice for many women to relieve the symptoms of menopause and PMS and to regulate any kind of menstrual dysfunction. Many people use it to enhance their sexual vitality.

Suggested uses: Vitex berries look and taste a bit like black pepper. Though they can be camouflaged in tea, they are most often used in tincture or capsule form.

Chickweed *(Stellaria media)*

Parts used: aerial parts

Benefits: Chickweed can be found worldwide in moist, cultivated soil, and is especially fond of gardens and yards. It is highly esteemed for its emollient and demulcent properties and is a major herb for skin irritations, eye inflammation, and kidney disorders. It is a mild diuretic and is indicated for water retention. It is an excellent poultice herb and is often found in salve formulas because of its soothing effects on the skin. In addition, it is a treasure trove of nutrients, including calcium, potassium, and iron.

Suggested uses: The fresh tender greens are delicious in salads. They can be juiced or blended with pineapple juice, and are often made into salves. And a light infusion of chickweed is quite soothing. The plant doesn't dry or store well, so to preserve it for future use, it is best to tincture it fresh.

Cleavers *(Galium aparine)*

Parts used: aerial parts of plant

Benefits: Another common garden weed, cleavers is often found growing near chickweed; the two are often combined in formulas. Both are mild, safe diuretics and both tone and soothe irritations of the kidneys and urinary tract. In addition, cleavers is an excellent lymphatic cleanser and is often used as a safe, effective remedy for swollen glands, tonsillitis, and some tumors.

Suggested uses: Prepare the same as chickweed. Cleavers also does not dry or store well, so prepare it as a tincture for future use.

Coltsfoot *(Tussilago farfara)*

Parts used: leaves

Benefits: So popular was coltsfoot in medieval days that it was chosen as the emblem to identify the local apothecary. Its botanical name, *Tussilago,* means "cough dispeller," and coltsfoot has long been cherished as a remedy for coughs, colds, and bronchial congestion. It is an antiasthmatic and expectorant, helping to dilate the bronchioles and expel mucus.

Suggested uses: Coltsfoot is often infused with other compatible lung herbs and served as a tea.

Caution: There is some concern about the safety of *Tussilago* because it has been found to contain PLAs, a harmful group of chemicals that can close off the veins to the liver. The studies have been inadequate and inconclusive. Since it has been used safely and effectively for hundreds of years, I continue to use it.

Comfrey *(Symphytum officinale)*

Parts used: leaves, roots

Benefits: Rich in allantoin and deeply healing, comfrey is used as a soothing poultice herb and in salves and ointments. It facilitates and activates the healing of tissue. It is one of the best herbs for torn ligaments, strains, bruises, and any injury to the bones or joints. Rich in mucilage, it soothes inflammation in the tissues when administered as a tea and in pills.

Suggested uses: The root and the leaf have similar properties; the root is stronger, the leaf is more palatable. Use them both in salves and ointments. The root is decocted, the leaf infused.

Caution: Comfrey was widely used in the '60s and '70s, but studies a few years ago found traces of PLAs (a group of toxic alkaloids that can cause a fatal liver disease). The studies were never conclusive and I'm so absolutely convinced that this herb is safe that I continue to use it personally, though I don't recommend it to others. You must make the choice for yourself.

Corn silk *(Zea mays)*

Part used: Golden, not brown, silk of organically grown corn

Benefits: The flower pistils from maize have long been used as a urinary tonic. It acts as an antiseptic, diuretic, and demulcent on the urinary system. It will stimulate and clean urinary passages while soothing inflammation.

Suggested uses: Corn silk is one of the most effective herbs for bed-wetting and incontinence. Use as a tea during the day to strengthen the urinary system. Take corn silk as a tincture at night to help prevent bed-wetting. Please note: Other treatments, such as kegel exercises, will have to be used in conjunction with corn silk for the treatment to be effective.

Dandelion *(Taraxacum officinale)*

Parts used: entire plant

Benefits: Half the world loves this plant, and uses it for medicine or dines on it daily. The other part of the population has been trying to destroy it with heavy chemical warfare since the 1940s. But dandelion's tenacity is part of its beauty and, perhaps, has something to do with its medicinal properties. The roots are a superior liver tonic. The leaves are a mild diuretic used for water retention and bladder or kidney problems. The flowers make a delicious wine, and the bitter greens of dandelion, rich in iron, calcium, and other trace minerals, are treasured the world over.

Suggested uses: Dandelion root is decocted and served as a tonic tea for the liver. The root, when tender, can be chopped like carrots and added to stir-fries and soups. The leaves are either infused for tea, steamed, or added raw to salads. Dandelion has a bitter zip to it, so it's best when blended with milder herbs. My favorite way to eat the leaves is to steam them, then marinate them overnight in Italian dressing and honey. Oh, my! This is good!

Echinacea (*Echinacea angustifolia*, *E. purpurea*, and related species)

Parts used: roots, leaves, flowers
Benefits: This beautiful, hearty plant is the best immune-enhancing herb that we know of and one of the most important herbs of our times. Though incredibly effective, it is not known to have any side effects or residual buildup in the body. Echinacea works by increasing macrophage T-cell activity, thereby increasing the body's first line of defense against colds, flus, and many other illnesses. Though potent and strong, it is 100 percent safe for even children to use.
Suggested uses: Take echinacea in frequent small doses in tea or tincture form to boost immunity at the first sign of a cold or flu. Useful for bronchial infections as a tea or tincture. Use as a spray for sore throats. For sore gums and mouth inflammation, make a mouthwash from the root and add peppermint or spearmint essential oil to flavor.
Caution: There are several types of echinacea available, but you should avoid wild-harvested varieties unless you know your source well. Because of the huge demand, echinacea is being poached mercilessly from its wild habitats.

Elder (*Sambucus nigra*)

Parts used: berries, flowers
Benefits: Elder flower syrup is Europe's most esteemed formula for colds, flus, and upper respiratory infections. Both the flowers and berries are powerful diaphoretics: by inducing sweating, they reduce fevers. Elder has immune-enhancing properties and is effectively combined with echinacea.
Suggested uses: Elderberries make some of the best syrups and wines you'll ever taste. The flowers are often used in teas for fever and are the main ingredient in elder flower water, a cosmetic wash. Every summer I collect the large, flat clusters of elder flowers and make a few fritters as a treat. They are delicious served with elderberry jam. There are several varieties of elder; use the variety that produces blue berries.

Elecampane *(Inula helenium)*

Parts used: roots

Benefits: A great sunflower-like plant, elecampane is easily grown in any garden. It is one of my favorite herbs for wet, mucus-type bronchial infections. As an expectorant and stimulating tonic, it is one of the best herbs for coughs, bronchitis, asthma, and chronic lung ailments.

Suggested uses: Elecampane is frequently combined with echinacea to combat deep-seated bronchial infections. The root is decocted. It also makes an effective tincture.

Fennel *(Foeniculum vulgare)*

Parts used: primarily seeds, but leaves and flowers are useful as well

Benefits: A well-known carminative and digestive aid, fennel was used by the early Greek physicians to increase and enrich the milk flow in nursing mothers. It is also an antacid, which both neutralizes excess acids in the stomach and intestines and clears uric acid from the joints. More generally, it stimulates digestion, regulates appetite, and relieves flatulence.

Suggested uses: A tasty fennel tea can be used for relieving colic, improving digestion, and expelling gas from the system. Nursing mothers can drink two to four cups daily to increase and enrich their flow of milk. Use a wash of warm fennel tea for conjunctivitis and other eye inflammations. Because of its delightful licorice-like taste, it's a useful flavoring agent.

HERBAL HISTORY

Our Puritan forefathers (and mothers!) used to mix carminitive (digestive-aiding) seeds such as anise, dill, fennel, and carway together. They would carry the mixture in little containers to the long church services. When the children's tummies growled from hunger or boredom, they would chew on these "meetin' seeds" to calm their stomachs.

Feverfew *(Tanacetum parthenium)*

Parts used: leaves, flowers

Benefits: This common garden flower has an outstanding reputation for the treatment of migraines. In 1772, an American herbalist wrote, "In the worst headache, this herb exceeds whatever else is known." Recent pharmacological studies have proven that it also alleviates inflammation and stress-related tension.

Suggested uses: As an infusion for managing migraines, drink the tea on a regular basis. I often combine it with lavender and use it in tincture form as a preventive for headaches and migraines. It is most effective for chronic migraines if taken over a period of one to three months, though it will also alleviate acute migraine symptoms.

Garlic *(Allium sativum)*

Parts used: bulbs

Benefits: Garlic is one of the oldest remedies known to humans. The sulfur and volatile oils in garlic make it a potent internal and external antiseptic. It stimulates the body's immune system to fight off infections. Garlic is a well-known vermifuge, used for expelling intestinal worms in humans and animals. It is very effective herb for maintaining healthy blood cholesterol levels and lowering high blood pressure. In addition to all of this, garlic is just plain tasty.

Suggested uses: Contrary to popular opinion, cooking garlic destroys little of its medicinal properties. According to the latest studies, the active ingredients may diminish a bit with cooking, but they are still present. Add garlic to your meals. It can be eaten raw by blending it in with pesto and dips. I tincture garlic, pickle it (with tamari and vinegar), and make herbal oils with it. It's among the most versatile of all herbs, willing to be used by all those who appreciate it.

Ginger *(Zingiber officinalis)*

Parts used: root

Benefits: A versatile and useful plant, ginger is used as both a culinary herb and a valuable medicinal plant. It is highly regarded as a primary herb for the reproductive, respiratory, and digestive systems. It is one of the main ingredients in reproductive tonics for men and women and helps improve poor circulation to the pelvis. It is a safe and often effective herb for motion sickness and morning sickness. It is my favorite remedy for cramps, and is a good diaphoretic that opens up the pores and promotes sweat. Ginger is a valued digestive aid, improving digestion and efficiently moving out waste.

Suggested uses: Ginger is rich in volatile oils and, although it's a root, is best infused. Grated ginger makes a delicious tea with lemon and honey. Ginger powder can be added to many formulas or used in cooking. Try making ginger syrup; it is simply delicious. Hot poultices of ginger applied over the pelvis helps with cramps and stomach tension.

Ginkgo *(Ginkgo biloba)*

Parts used: leaves, fruit

Benefits: One of my favorite plants, ginkgo is the sole survivor of the oldest known tree genus, *Ginkgoaceae,* which dates back over 200 million years. This is one of the best memory aids, vitality enhancers, and circulatory herbs. I suggest it as a regular tonic herb for everybody over 45. In recent studies, it has been shown to halt the process of Alzheimer's when administered in therapeutic dosages over a period of time. Ginkgo must be used with consistency for several weeks or months before one notices its benefits.

Suggested uses: Use the standardized capsules or extracts when treating Alzheimer's disease. To strengthen the mind and for circulation, ginkgo is effective served as a tea or in tincture or capsules.

Goldenseal (Hydrastis canadensis)

Part used: roots, leaves

Benefits: This is quite possibly one of the most useful and valuable plants of North America. Particularly effective at healing mucous membranes, goldenseal is used in cleansing washes for the eye, as a douche for infections (careful: it can be too drying for the vagina if not formulated correctly), in mouthwashes for sore mouths and gums, and in the topical treatment of eczema and psoriasis. It is a natural antibiotic and is often combined with echinacea to help fight infections and ward off colds and flus.

Suggested uses: Goldenseal is strongly bitter and is often used as a bitter tonic and digestive aid. The root is infused (not decocted) as a bitter tea, and used as a mouthwash for gum infections and a wash for cuts. It is often powdered and used in poultices for infections, abscesses, and wounds. Combine with echinacea to help fight off infections and colds.

Caution: Use only organically cultivated varieties of this endangered plant, or grow your own if you have woodlands. If used over a period of time, goldenseal becomes an irritant to the mucous membranes, causing inflammation and irritation. Always rotate its use and do not take for longer than three weeks at a time.

Hawthorn (Crataegus species)

Parts used: fruits, flowers, leaves

Benefits: This is the best heart tonic herb there is. It has been revered and surrounded by legend for centuries. Hawthorn dilates the arteries and veins, allowing blood to flow more freely and releasing cardiovascular constrictions and blockages. It lowers blood pressure while strengthening the heart muscle. It also helps maintain healthy cholesterol levels. Hawthorn is outstanding both to prevent heart problems and to treat heart disease, edema, angina, and heart arrhythmia.

Suggested uses: Delicious as a tea, syrup, and jam, hawthorn can also be tinctured. Use on a regular basis.

Hibiscus (*Hibiscus sabdariff* and related species)

Parts used: flowers
Benefits: Hibiscus is high in vitamin C and bioflavonoids. It has slightly astringent properties and a rich, beautiful color.
Suggested uses: This is the plant that made Celestial Seasonings famous. The large tropical flowers make a bright red tea that is tart, with a sweet aftertaste. I'll often formulate hibiscus with stevia or other sweet herbs to enhance the flavor.

Lavender (*Lavandula* species)

Parts used: flowers
Benefits: Native to the Mediterranean, lavender blesses us with a range of uses. Beautiful, fragrant, and hardy, it is a strong nervine, a mild antidepressant, and an aid for headaches. Combined with feverfew, it helps alleviate migraines. It is one of the best herbs to add to the bath for alleviating tension, stress, and insomnia. The oil is excellent for insect bites, bee stings, and burns (mix with honey).
Suggested uses: Add small amounts to tea (its flavor can be overpowering). It makes a tasty glycerin- or alcohol-based tincture. The essential oil is used in bathwater and can be inhaled to soothe the nerves. For headaches, apply two to three drops to temples and nape of neck. Apply topically for insect bites. Use as a wash for cuts, or in a bath, salve, or steam to relieve congestion.

HERB TIP

Lavender oil has been called "a first-aid kit in a bottle," and can be used effectively for a number of situations. When my student, Lila, and I were working together in the gardens she knelt upon a bee. The poor, unsuspecting creature stung her quite ferociously. But Lila pulled out a bottle of lavender oil from her pocket and applied a few dabs to the wound. The area hardly swelled and she reported very little pain.

Lemon balm (Melissa officinalis)

Parts used: leaves

Benefits: Calming, antiviral, and antiseptic, this beautifully fragrant member of the mint family is one of nature's best nervine herbs. Applied topically, it has been found to be helpful for herpes. It is often made into a cream for this purpose, though I find the tincture works as well. Lemon balm tea is used as a mild sedative and for insomnia.

Suggested uses: Lemon balm makes a delicious tea and can be served with lemon and honey throughout the day to alleviate stress and anxiety. For a delicious nervine tonic, blend equal amounts of lemon balm, oats, and chamomile. Lemon balm makes one of the tastiest tinctures, in either alcohol or glycerin.

Licorice (Glycyrrhiza glabra)

Parts used: roots

Benefits: The effective yet delicious qualities of licorice help make it one of our most important herbal remedies. It is used for a multitude of situations, including bronchial congestion, sore throat, and coughs, and helps to heal inflammations of the digestive tract such as ulcers or nonspecific sores. It is excellent for toning the endocrine system and is a specific for adrenal exhaustion. It is a favorite herb of singers for strengthening their voices. Licorice is one of the most widely used herbs in the world, yet it is a humble, little plant, well sheathed in a woody exterior that hides its inherent sweetness.

Suggested uses: Licorice is almost sickeningly sweet and must be blended with other herbs to be palatable. Use in syrups, teas, and tinctures and as an herbal wash. Children often enjoy chewing on licorice sticks.

Marsh mallow
(Althaea officinalis)

Parts used: primarily roots, but leaves and flowers are useful
Benefits: A soothing, mucilaginous herb, marsh mallow can be used similarly to slippery elm, but is much more readily available and easy to grow in most garden settings.
Suggested uses: Serve as a tea for sore throats, diarrhea, constipation, and bronchial inflammation. Mix into a paste with water for soothing irritated skin. Marsh mallow can also be used in the bath along with oatmeal for a soothing wash.

Milk thistle (Silybum marianum)

Parts used: seeds, leaves
Benefits: The seeds of this large wild thistle are nature's best aid for damaged liver tissue. In fact, it is even used in allopathic medicine and is the only agent known to prevent fatal amanita (death cap mushroom) poisoning. It directly stimulates liver function and rebuilds damaged liver tissues. Its tonifying actions make it a valuable component of cleansing programs and an important supplement for those whose livers have been compromised by illness, hepatitis, or alcohol consumption. Milk thistle seed is also helpful for the gallbladder and the kidneys.
Suggested uses: The hard black seeds should be ground in a coffee mill so that the chemical constituents can be more easily drawn out. Use in tinctures or tea, or sprinkle directly on food (the seeds are tasty).

Motherwort *(Leonurus cardiaca)*

Parts used: leaves

Benefits: Motherwort is best known for its beneficial properties for women, especially for menopausal women, but it's equally beneficial as a heart tonic. Its botanical name, *Leonurus,* means lionhearted. It is a superb tonic for nourishing and strengthening the heart muscle and its blood vessels. It is a remedy for most heart disease, neuralgia, and an over-rapid heartbeat. It is valued for many women's problems, including delayed menstruation, uterine cramps associated with scanty menses, water retention, and hot flashes and mood swings during menopause.

Motherwort grows easily in the garden. It is weedlike, so be careful! In addition, motherwort often is found growing in the wild.

Suggested uses: Serve several times a day as an infusion flavored with tastier herbs and as a tincture.

Mullein *(Verbascum thapsus)*

Parts used: leaves, flowers, roots

Benefits: This is one of my favorite wayside weeds. It is always so stately, sending its flowering stalk sometimes several feet into the sky. That stalk is full of beautiful, fragrant yellow flowers that make the "world's best oil" for ear infections. Mullein used to be called torch plant or candlestick plant because its long, flowering stalks were dried, dipped in fat or oil, and lit as a slow-burning torch.

The leaves are used most often and are employed in cough formulas and used for respiratory infections, bronchial infections, and asthma. The leaves are excellent for treating glandular imbalances.

Suggested uses: The flowers are generally made into oil for the ears. The leaves are either used as a tincture or an infusion for bronchial congestion, colds, and coughs. For glandular problems, mix with echinacea and cleavers.

Nettle *(Urtica dioica)*

Parts used: fresh leaves, young tops

Benefits: Nettle is high in vitamins and minerals, especially iron and calcium. It is an excellent remedy for allergies and hay fever, and useful for growing pains in young children, when their bones and joints ache (just like older folks!). An excellent reproductive tonic for men and women, nettle is used for alleviating the symptoms of PMS and menopause. One of my favorite all-around remedies, it also makes a great hair and scalp tonic.

Suggested uses: Nettle is a pleasant-tasting food and is often steamed and served as a calcium- and iron-rich addition to meals. It can be used to replace spinach in any recipe, but must always be well steamed; it will sting you if undercooked! It is delicious as a tea and can be served several times a day to prevent allergic attacks. Freeze-dried nettle capsules have the best reputation for treating allergies and hay fever, but I often combine the capsules with tea.

Oats *(Avena sativa)*

Parts used: green milky tops, but stems are useful

Benefits: One of the best nutritive tonics for the nervous system, oats are recommended for nervous exhaustion, stress, and irritation. The plant's mucilaginous properties make it particularly helpful for damage to the myelin sheath. Oats are high in silica and calcium.

Suggested uses: Best used partially green, before the plant has turned golden. Both the milky green tops and the stalks make a delicious tea — one of the best, I think. Make it strong and mix with fruit juice. Used for people who are nervous, hyperactive, or stressed, it also makes a wonderfully soothing bath for skin irritations.

Oregon grape *(Mahonia aquafolium)*

Parts used: roots

Benefits: The roots of this beautiful hollylike plant are gaining fame — hopefully not to its demise — because it contains berberine, a compound similar to that found in goldenseal. There's some indication that it can be used in place of goldenseal to help prevent overharvesting of that herb, but Oregon grape is a slow-growing perennial with a limited growing range. It is a good herb used to fight systemic infection as well as for topical cleansing. By restoring equilibrium, it can cure skin problems such as acne, eczema, and psoriasis.

Suggested uses: The decocted root can be used as a topical wash for infections, or taken internally. Oregon grape root has exceptional anti-inflammatory, antiseptic, and antiviral properties. Take internally for infections, poor digestion, and as a tonic for the liver.

Caution: Be careful of overharvesting in the wild. Though often prolific where it is found growing, Oregon grape has limited range. We may determine this herb should be used from cultivated sources and leave the wild stands to grow.

Passionflower *(Passiflora incarnata)*

Parts used: leaves, flowers

Benefits: This is certainly one of the best herbs for calming the nervous system, contrary to what its name implies. Passionflower is used for stress, anxiety, and depression. An effective, gentle herb, it can be used for hyperactive children as well as adults.

Suggested uses: The leaves and flowers are brewed as an infusion and the tea drunk throughout the day. Use the tincture at bedtime to aid in peaceful sleep.

Peppermint *(Mentha x piperita)*

Parts used: leaves, flowers

Benefits: Peppermint has often been called "a blast of pure green energy." It's not that there aren't stronger stimulants, but none that makes you feel so renewed and refreshed. Commonly used as a digestive aid, peppermint is effective for treating nausea, easing stomach cramps, and clearing the mouth of foul tastes. It's a common ingredient in toothpastes and tooth powders.

Suggested uses: Use for sluggish digestion and a burst of "green energy." Use peppermint in tea or diluted tincture as a mouthwash. Because of its pleasant and familiar flavor, peppermint is often used to flavor less tasty herbs. It is purely delicious fresh from the garden.

Plantain *(Plantago major, P. lanceolata)*

Parts used: seeds, roots, leaves

Benefits: Plantain is easily found and is a highly nutritional food. It is one of the best poultice herbs and is often referred to as the Green Bandage. It's among my favorite herbs for treating blood poisoning, used externally on the infected area and internally as a tea. The plantain seeds are rich in mucilage and are often used in laxative blends for their soothing bulk action. In fact, psyllium seeds used in Metamucil are produced from a *Plantago* species. This herb is also very effective for treating liver sluggishness and inflammation of the digestive tract.

Suggested uses: Though it is often considered a bitter, plantain is quite mild in flavor and makes a nice infusion. See directions on page 13 for a plantain poultice. It can also be powdered and added to food or used as an herbal first-aid powder for infections.

Red clover *(Trifolium pratense)*

Parts used: flowering tops, leaves

Benefits: Red clover is one of the best respiratory tonics for young children, and is one of the best detoxification herbs. It is used for chronic chest complaints such as coughs, colds, and bronchitis. It is rich in nitrogen and minerals, most notably calcium and iron. It is used for all skin conditions and commonly used in antitumor formulas.

Suggested uses: Red clover makes a delicious tea. Blend with other herbs such as mullein for persistent respiratory problems. Use as a tea for building blood and improving the skin. The tea or tincture can be used for growths on the body such as cysts, tumors, and fibroids.

Caution: Do not use consistently for hemophiliacs or people with "thin" blood, as it can promote bleeding.

Red raspberry *(Rubus idaeus)*

Parts used: young shoots, fruits, and leaves

Benefits: Raspberry was first cited in Chinese herbal writings dating back to A.D. 550, and was a valuable remedy to the native peoples of the North American continent. It has been used as a uterine tonic and nutritive supplement ever since. Raspberry leaves are rich in vitamins and minerals, particularly calcium and iron.

Suggested uses: As a tea or tincture, raspberry leaf is valuable for treating diarrhea and dysentery. It helps reduce excessive menstruation and is one of the superior tonics for pregnancy and childbirth. Because of its astringent properties, it is a good mouthwash for sore or infected gums.

ROSE HIPS JAM

Dried rose hips make a delicious jam, but be sure they're seedless. Cover with fresh apple juice; soak overnight. The next day the jam is ready to eat. You can add cinnamon and other spices, but it's good enough to eat as is.

Rose hips (Rosa canina and related species)

Parts used: primarily seeds, but leaves and flowers are useful
Benefits: Rose hips contain more vitamin C than almost any other herb, many times that of citrus fruit when measured gram by gram. Vitamin C is a noted antioxidant with disease-fighting capabilities. Rose leaves are astringent and toning. The flowers are used in love potions and flower essences.
Suggested uses: Make fresh rose hips into a vitamin-rich syrup or jam. Rose hips make a delicious, mild-flavored tea, perfect on a cold New England night, sipped by a roaring fire.

Rosemary (Rosmarinus officinalis)

Parts used: leaves
Benefits: I think we've only begun to uncover the many uses of rosemary. It has long been renowned as a memory aid and as a symbol of remembrance. It has a tonic effect on the nervous system and is good for circulation. It strengthens the heart and reduces high blood pressure. It has been used for hundreds of years as a cosmetic herb for its effects on the hair and skin.
Suggested uses: Blended with other herbs in the famous Queen of Hungary's Water, rosemary is part of a bracing astringent cosmetic preparation. It makes a pleasant tea when infused with other herbs and is often blended with ginkgo and gota kola in tincture and tea form as a memory aid.

Sage (Salvia officinalis)

Parts used: leaves

Benefits: Warming and strengthening, sage is a courageous fellow. Even its name, *Salvia,* means to save. It is an excellent herb for rebuilding vitality and strength during long-term illness. It clears congestion and soothes sore throats, tonsillitis, and laryngitis.

Suggested uses: Make into a gargle for sore throat and infections in the mouth. An infusion of sage is pleasant and warming. Perhaps because of its grounding nature, sage is helpful for menopausal women, most specifically for hot flashes. Of course, sage is excellent as a culinary herb and enhances the flavor of many foods.

St.-John's-wort (Hypericum perforatum and related species)

Parts used: leaves, flowers

Benefits: This, along with echinacea, has become another "pin up" herb. Although it has been used for centuries for nerve damage and has always been held in high esteem by herbalists, it was recently "discovered" for its antidepressant activities. It is a wonderfully safe and effective herb for nerve damage, stress, anxiety, depression, and personality disorders. The beautiful red oil made magically from the cheerful yellow flowers is a wonderful "trauma" oil, used for bruises, sprains, burns, and injuries of all kinds.

Suggested uses: Definitely make St.-John's-wort oil; it is one of the finest medicinal oils. The herb is best used fresh, though I have seen some outstanding dried plant material that seems to be highly effective. The flowers and leaves are tinctured or prepared as an infusion (use approximately 70 percent flower to 30 percent leaf). Though some people claim St.-John's-wort causes sensitivity to the sun, many people use it in sunscreen to protect them from burning. I wonder if sun sensitivity is enhanced by stress and anxiety?

Caution: St.-John's-wort does cause photosensitivy in some individuals. There was some earlier concern that St.-John's-wort worked similarly to Prozac as an MAO inhibitor, but this is not true. The action of St.-John's-wort is not completely understood, but it is not an MAO inhibitor and, therefore, the restrictions imposed on Prozac users do not apply to those taking St.-John's-wort.

Saw palmetto *(Serenoa repens)*

Parts used: berries
Benefits: This is the herb supreme for men, and has gained great popularity in recent years. Even doctors recommend it to their male patients as a tonic and preventive herb, as well as a specific remedy for enlarged prostate glands. Not so well known are its benefits for women. It firms sagging breast tissue and is an excellent herb for those who are thin and are unable to gain weight.
Suggested uses: The berries are quite pungent and strong tasting; nothing seems to mask their rather unpleasant taste. Because of its flavor, saw palmetto is used primarily in tinctures and capsules.

Siberian ginseng *(Eleuthero-coccus senticosus)*

Parts used: roots
Benefits: Also known as eleuthero, more than 1,000 scientific studies have confirmed this herb's remarkable properties for enhancing physical and mental performance. Although it is not botanically related to ginseng, it is commonly called Siberian ginseng because of its adaptogenic properties and similarity to ginseng. It strengthens the nervous, endocrine, and immune systems.

Suggested uses: Use as a long-term tonic. The powdered herbs are added to pills and tonic recipes. The root is decocted as a tea. The chopped dry root can also be added to soup. (Remove the chunks before eating; they stay hard.)

Slippery elm (Ulmus fulva)

Parts used: inner bark

Benefits: A soothing mucilaginous herb, slippery elm is one of the most beloved of medicinal herbs. However, the elm trees of America have been severely depleted due to Dutch elm disease. Use sparingly.

Suggested uses: Slippery elm is used for soothing any and all inflammations, whether internal or external. It is particularly valuable for burns, sore throats, and digestive problems, including diarrhea and constipation. A highly nourishing food, it was at one time sold as a medicinal flour and used in cooking and baking.

Caution: Be selective when using this herb. Whenever possible, use marsh mallow externally as a substitute for it. When you do purchase it, know your source and buy only from ethical harvesters who gather bark from limbs of fallen trees or who use farm-grown slippery elm.

Spearmint (Mentha spicata)

Parts used: leaves, flowers

Benefits: Cooling, refreshing, uplifting, spearmint is one of the most popular of all the mints. It has a cool, refreshing flavor. You can use spearmint to lift the flavors of other less tasty herbs.

Suggested uses: Use to "sweeten" the stomach and breath after sickness, especially vomiting. Add a drop of the essential oil to water, or make a cup of fresh tea, and rinse the mouth out several times. Add to uplifting, refreshing herb blends, to honey, and to food for a flavorful, quick pick-me-up. Of course, spearmint is the herb of choice in the dental industry.

Stevia *(Stevia rebundiana)*

Parts used: leaves

Benefits: Called the sweet herb, stevia is sweeter than sugar but much better for you. It has no calories and doesn't promote tooth decay. It is indicated for pancreatic imbalances and high blood sugar levels, and is a type of sugar that diabetics can tolerate. In fact, stevia has been used to help treat diabetes. Though stevia has been tested extensively in other countries, it was banned in the United States on the pretext that its safety was unknown. Now that several of the large sugar companies have secured an interest in stevia production, the herb quite suddenly has been legalized in the United States.

Suggested uses: Because of its intense sweetness, stevia is primarily used to enhance the flavor of other herbs. The only problem is that it is far too sweet. If you add even a pinch too much to a cup of tea or a recipe, you'll ruin the flavor.

Usnea *(Usnea barbata)*

Parts used: lichens

Benefits: It is odd that an herb so abundant and so useful was not used by modern American herbalists until just a few years ago. Usnea is the lichen that grows on primarily aging trees and is often called "old man's beard"; since several lichens are called by this name, be sure the one you are using is usnea. Containing the bitter principle usnic acid, usnea soothes the stomach while enhancing digestion. It has antibiotic properties, making it useful for treating urinary and bladder infections, cystitis, and fungal infections. It is an excellent immune enchancer and is frequently combined with echinacea.

Suggested uses: I often add a small amount of usnea to soup. It is easily powdered and mixed with foods or blended into capsules; however, its taste leaves something to be desired. Usnea is most often tinctured, as its seems most effective in an alcohol solvent.

Uva ursi (Arctostaphylos uva-ursi)

Parts used: leaves, berries

Benefits: Uva ursi is a small, wiry shrub that hugs the earth. Its leatherlike leaves are harvested and used as tea for kidney and bladder infections. It is an effective diuretic, astringent, and urinary antiseptic that cleans and heals urinary passages. It is used for cystitis, urethritis, kidney stones, leukorrhea, and bed-wetting.

Suggested uses: Uva ursi is most effective as an infusion used for inflammation and infection. However, a decoction will bring out a richer concentration of tannins and the plant's astringent properties. Uva ursi is often infused as a strong tea and mixed with cranberry juice for bladder and kidney infections.

Valerian (Valeriana officinalis)

Parts used: roots

Benefits: This is one of my favorite nerve tonics and muscle relaxants. For those people whom valerian works for, it works well. Some people, however, find it irritating and overly stimulating. It is effective for insomnia, pain, restlessness, headaches, digestive problems due to nerves, and muscle spasms. Depending on the individual, the smell is either relished or deemed offensive. I rather love the odor, which reminds people of violets, rich sweet earth, or dirty underwear, depending on the age of the root.

Suggested uses: Because the root is rich in volatile oils, it should be infused rather than decocted. Valerian is often tinctured or encapsulated rather than taken as tea because of its odor, though its taste is quite pleasant. Herbalists are in disagreement about whether the fresh or dried herb works better. Without a doubt, it's better tasting when fresh. Cats love it, often better than catnip.

White oak *(Quercus alba)*

Parts used: bark

Benefits: The white oak is a huge, stately tree, whose bark is a powerful astringent and disinfectant. Its high tannin content makes it useful for treating diarrhea and hemorrhoids, as an astringent antiseptic wash for wounds, poison oak, and poison ivy, and as a gargle for sore throats and mouth infections. It is a good remedy for leukorreha (a common vaginal discharge often called "the whites") and varicose veins.

Suggested uses: Commonly made into a decoction for internal purposes and an antiseptic liniment for external purposes, white oak also tinctures well, and is often found in formulas for sore throats and infections.

Wild cherry *(Prunus serotina)*

Parts used: inner bark

Benefits: One of the best herbs for coughs, wild cherry is a pectoral expectorant calming most types of coughs. It is one of the few herbs still included in the United States Pharmacopeia and it is still found in some commercial cough remedies.

Suggested uses: Wild cherry is a favorite herb to include in teas, syrups, and tinctures for coughs and colds. It is also a digestive bitter that improves digestion and promotes healthy bowel function.

HARVESTING FROM "GRANDFATHER TREE"

Shortly after I moved to New England, one of my large wild cherry trees crashed down in the aftermath of a winter storm. By afternoon's ebb my grandson and I had collected enough bark to give away to friends and still make the best cough syrup ever. Andrew still asks for Wild Cherry Syrup from "Grandfather Tree."

Wild yam (Dioscorea villosa)

Parts used: roots

Benefits: Wild yam has a complex action on the body and is used for a variety of important purposes. It is a primary source material for steroid production and is a hormone precursor. It normalizes the function of the endocrine glands and aids in the normal function of the reproductive system of both sexes. I have used it successfully to treat all aspects of menstrual dysfunction and to help people increase fertility, although I have heard of people who use it as a "natural" form of birth control. It is also a nervine and antispasmodic and is excellent for soothing muscle cramps, colic, and uterine pain. It is also useful for liver congestion and gallbladder function.

Suggested uses: Use wild yam in formulas for the reproductive system of men and women. It can be made into teas, tinctures, and capsules.

Caution: This plant is listed on the United Plant Savers "at-risk" list. It is severely depleted in its natural habitats. Buy only from organic sources.

Witch hazel (Hamamelis virginiana)

Parts used: bark

Benefits: A North American shrub, witch hazel was being used by the natives when European settlers first arrived. It is a potent pain reliever and astringent. It is thought to act on the venous system to stop bleeding and inflammation both internally and externally. It is particularly effective for intestinal bleeding, hemorrhoids, varicose veins, and diarrhea. It is also indicated for bleeding of the nose and lungs.

Suggested uses: Witch hazel is often made into a tincture or liniment and used externally as an astringent, disinfectant wash. It also makes a good cleanser for "troubled" skin. Decocted as tea, it is used internally as an astringent for diarrhea and intestinal bleeding.

Yarrow *(Achillea millefolium* and related wild species)

Parts used: leaves, flowers

Benefits: A beautiful roadside weed, yarrow is best recognized by its creamy flowers that bloom throughout the summer months. It is an excellent diaphoretic, often used in teas to promote sweating, thereby helping to reduce fevers. Yarrow is an old first-aid item used to stop bleeding both internally and externally. It is effective for both menstrual and stomach cramps and is often used in formulas for stomach flus. It also has beneficial effects on the heart and lungs.

Suggested uses: Yarrow makes a bitter infusion, so blend with tastier herbs as a digestive aid and diaphoretic. The dried, powdered leaves are useful first-aid items for wounds and cuts, both disinfecting the wounds and helping to stop bleeding. A pinch of the powder can be placed in the nose to stop a nosebleed.

Yellow dock *(Rumex crispus)*

Parts used: roots

Benefits: This abundant wild weed of fields, gardens, and roadsides is quite possibly one of the best herbs for the entire digestive system, including the liver. The large taproot is rich in anthraquinone, which has a laxative action. It is an easily digested form of biochelated iron that can readily be absorbed. It is one of the best herbs for anemia and fatigue, and is useful for women with PMS and men and women with hormonal problems.

Suggested uses: The chemical constituents are readily extracted by a water decoction and by alcohol. Yellow dock makes a somewhat bitter tasting decoction so is best formulated with more flavorful herbs. It makes a good tincture for the liver, gallbladder, and aids digestion. It can be added to formulas for its laxative properties. I've also made iron-rich syrups with the root.

chapter four

Making Your Own First-Aid Kit

Y ou may find, as many others have, that herbs become a passion. Slowly but surely, they take over the entire house; first it's only a small space in the bathroom closet, then a cupboard in the kitchen is cleared, next the entire basement is given over to your herbal wares, and the cars are parked in the driveway because the garage is filled with bottles of odd-looking preparations. About this time your family may be saying, "no more." But let's assume you're a long way from there and you just want to organize a small kit of useful herbal remedies.

What Do I Need?

To make an herbal first-aid kit, assess the needs of yourself and your family, and the situations that may arise requiring first aid. Do you have young children? What maladies is your family prone to? A good kit consists of items that can be used for a variety of purposes.

Keep your herbal first-aid kit in one place so it's readily available to you and your family. Baskets, sewing boxes, small suitcases, travel pouches, cosmetic bags, and fishing tackle boxes make great containers for first-aid kits. Be sure everything is clearly labeled so that others can use it.

First Aid in the Backyard

Everywhere, under every footstep, along the roadsides, in empty city lots, in country fields, and thriving beneath the pavement of superhighways, one can find valuable medicinal herbs. One would be foolish not to discover the wealth of medicinals growing in the backyard. These plants thrive in most regions (except tropical zones) in the United States and are found in abundance. You'll find a short description on each in chapter 3.

Make friends with these plants:

- Plantain
- Dandelion
- Self-heal
- Burdock
- Chickweed
- Nettle
- Yellow dock
- Cleavers
- Yarrow
- Red Clover
- Wild Raspberry
- Mullein
- Coltsfoot
- St.-John's-wort

What's in the Kitchen

Many of my favorite medicinal plants have sneaked into the household via the kitchen door, ushered in by the Mistress of Spices, their healing spirits camouflaged in culinary garb. Most of your favorite kitchen herbs are renowned healers, respected throughout the ages by various cultures. Many are still found in very effective remedies and even pharmaceutical preparations.

Basil

A favorite tonic for melancholy and low spirits, basil's antispasmodic properties make it useful for headaches. It is commonly used to treat stress-induced insomnia and tension, nervous indigestion, and is a well-known aphrodisiac.

Black Pepper

Considered one of the great tonics in traditional Chinese medicine, black pepper is warming, energizing, and stimulating. It is indicated for "cold type" problems such as flus, coughs, colds, slow circulation, and poor digestion. Some people find it an irritant; Jethro Kloss, a famous herbalist of the early 1900s, publicized it as a toxic substance. However, most people tolerate it well.

Cardamom

A divinely sensual flavor, cardamom belongs to the same family as ginger. It stimulates the mind and arouses the senses. It has long been considered an aphrodisiac, in part because of its irresistible flavor. In Ayurvedic medicine, cardamom is considered one of the best digestive aids. It is often combined as an anticatarrhal in formulas for the lungs.

First-aid Kit Items

Lots of herbs work well for minor emergencies. In addition to your favorite medicinal teas, stock an assortment of powdered herbs for different purposes; they are easy to mix for poultices and to encapsulate as needed.

ITEM	FORM	USE FOR
All-purpose/ burn salve	salve	cuts, wounds, burns, sunburns
Aloe vera	gel	burns, wounds, and cuts
Antifungal salve	salve	cuts, wounds, burns, sunburns
Cold care capsules	capsules	colds, sluggish digestion, infections
Echinacea	tincture	immune enhancer, colds, flus, infections
Eucalyptus	essential oil	congestion (added to steams), achy muscles, insect repellent, cuts and abrasions, warts, cold sores
Garlic	oil	ear infections, parasites, colds
Green clay	powder	splinters, wound disinfectant, poultices for poison oak/ivy, skin infections
Kloss's liniment	tincture/ liniment	splinters and slivers, poison oak/ivy. For external use only. See recipe on page 68.
Lavender	essential oil	headaches, minor burns and sunburn, insect bites, congestion
Licorice root	tincture	sore throats, bronchial inflammation, herpes simplex I & II
Mullein flower	oil	ear infections, pain
Peppermint	essential oil	digestive problems, burns, mouthwash, stimulant
Rescue Remedy	flower essence	trauma, both emotional and physical; can be used externally and internally for adults, children, and pets
St.-John's-wort	oil	burns, swellings, pain, bruises, sunburn, achy muscles
St.-John's-wort	tincture	burns, pain, nerve damage, depression, anxiety
Tea Tree	oil	*see* eucalyptus, also good for toothaches
Valerian	tincture	pain, insomnia, stress and nervous tension, achy muscles

Cayenne

This herb is as esteemed for its medicinal value as for its culinary fire. It is a supreme heart tonic and has long been used for poor circulation and for irregular or weak heartbeat. It is specifically indicated for colds and flus, used to increase circulation to the extremities, and to improve digestion and sluggish bowels. It is also used internally and externally to halt bleeding.

Chives

Similar to garlic, though not as potent, chives have the same antiseptic properties as garlic. It helps in the digestion of rich foods and protects the respiratory system. People sensitive to garlic can often enjoy the medicinal and culinary benefits of chives.

Cinnamon

Highly valued in traditional Chinese medicine as a warming and stimulating herb, cinnamon is used to raise vitality, stimulate circulation, and clear congestion. It is a well-respected digestive aid and has powerful antiseptic actions as well. Indicated for poor digestion, colds, and flus, cinnamon is often used in medicinal formulas to flavor the less tasty herbs.

Cloves

Clove oil is most famous as an analgesic herb for toothaches, but the entire clove bud, powdered and applied directly to the gum, is as effective. Aside from its analgesic properties, clove is stimulating, warming, and uplifting. It is used for sluggish digestion and nausea.

Dill

Dill is one of the most famous of old English remedies for infant colic. Nursery songs were made up about it and sung to the children. Dill's warming and comforting qualities are indicated for gas and colicky digestion. It's also an old folk remedy for hiccups.

Garlic

Were I forced to have only one herb in my kitchen, garlic would be it. There's nothing that enhances the flavor of foods or improves health more than garlic. It is the herb of choice for colds, flus, sore throats, and poor digestion. It stimulates immune activity, improves circulation, and lowers cholesterol. It has a long reputation as a culinary herb and an even longer reputation as a medicinal plant. Garlic, the infamous "stinking rose," may be nothing less than one of the world's greatest medicines.

Ginger

Ginger runs a close second to garlic in my estimation. It is one of the finest herbs for nausea, morning sickness, and motion sickness. Ginger is a warming, decongesting herb used for cold-type imbalances such as poor circulation, sore throats, colds, flus, and congestion. It is a wonderful herb for the reproductive systems of men and women, often used in formulas for cramps and PMS. And if that wasn't enough, it is quite delicious and used to flavor less tasty medicinal herbs.

Horseradish

What better natural remedy is there for sinus congestion and head colds? This is my number one favorite. The root is rich in minerals, including silica, and rich in vitamins, including vitamin C. Its warming antiseptic properties make it the herb of choice for asthma, catarrh, and lung infections. Horseradish is also prized as a digestive aid and is especially useful when eating heavy, hard to digest meals.

Marjoram and Oregano

Calming and soothing herbs, both marjoram and oregano are used for nervousness, irritability, and insomnia due to tension and anxiety. Great to drink as a tea — either in combination or singly — when feeling edgy or to calm butterflies in the stomach. These delicious herbs also have antispasmodic properties that can be used advantageously for digestive and muscular spasms.

Mint (Peppermint, Spearmint, and Lemon Balm)

Rich in vitamin C, beta carotene, and chlorophyll, mints are stimulating to the mind and create "wakefulness." Whiffs of the essential oil, sometimes even the tea, will improve alertness and awareness, so it's useful when driving, studying, and during times of stress. It is an excellent antispasmodic and is indicated for cramps and spasms. A terrific remedy for nausea, mint is recommended for travel sickness and some cases of morning sickness. It's also great for tummy aches in children and adults. The flavor of mint cleanses the palate and can be used to rinse the mouth after a bout of vomiting.

Parsley

This superb garnish should never be left slighted on the side of a platter. It may be, in fact, the most nourishing item on your dinner plate. High in iron, beta carotene, and chlorophyll, parsley is used for iron-poor blood, anemia, and fatigue. It will enhance immunity and is indicated when one is prone to infections. A primary herb for bladder and kidney problems, it is a safe, effective diuretic. Parsley is used for helping to dry up a mother's milk during the weaning process and is effective as a poultice for mastitis or swollen, enlarged breasts. Because of this, you should not use parsley in any quantities when nursing as it may slow the flow of milk.

Rocket (Arugula)

Imagine my delight when I discovered that arugula, my favorite salad green, was a famous sexual stimulant and tonic. I'm not sure whether to indulge more or be more temperate in my servings.

Rosemary

As this is my namesake, I must admit that I have some preference for this herb. The herb is legendary as a cerebral tonic and stimulant to the brain. Powerful for those states of debility that are accompanied by loss of memory, loss of smell, poor vision, strain, and nervous tension, rosemary also enhances the cellular uptake of oxygen. It is useful for relieving respiratory congestion and for maintaining liver function and digestion.

Sage

There's an old saying that where rosemary thrives in the garden, the woman rules the house, but where sage thrives, the man rules. Sage is another remarkable culinary remedy. It aids in the digestion of fatty meats, lowers cholesterol levels, and is a tonic for the liver. It has antiseptic properties and helps with colds, sore throats, and ear infections. It is one of the best remedies for laryngitis and sore throats, often used as a spray or gargle.

Thyme

This is the best herb we have for stimulating the thymus, a major gland of the immune system. Thyme is a great pick-me-up for low energy. Its antispasmodic properties are useful for lung problems and for convulsive coughs such as whooping cough. It's an excellent remedy for sore throats (combined with sage), head colds (combined with horseradish), and stiffness related to chills. Thyme also helps stimulate the body's natural defense and, combined with echinacea, boosts the immune system.

Turmeric

This is one of the best herbs for immune health and is often overlooked because of the huge popularity of echinacea. But it has upheld its reputation for its immune-enhancing properties for centuries and is highly regarded for its antitumor and antibiotic activities. In East Indian medicine, it is valued as a blood purifier and metabolic tonic. It is used to regulate the menstrual cycle and relieve cramps, reduce fevers, improve poor circulation, and relieve skin disorders. It is highly valued as a first-aid item for boils, burns, sprains, swelling, and bruises.

chapter five

Simple and Effective Household Remedies

I n the past, common, everyday ailments were treated either by someone in the family or by the local healer or herbalist. Many of these problems respond well to herbal treatment. I have included several common maladies here, along with favorite suggestions and time-tested recipes for effective herbal medicines. If your situation does not respond to these safe and simple suggestions, seek the help of a healthcare professional, ideally one knowledgeable about natural remedies.

Athlete's Foot

Athlete's foot is a fungal infection of the feet. Often itchy, it can spread to the hands. In dealing with athlete's foot, it is important to keep feet dry, socks clean, and to go shoeless or wear sandles as much as possible to air your feet.

Several treatments are available for this common infection. Try sprinkling tea tree oil directly on the area that is infected. Soak the feet several nights a week in a hot footbath with chaparral and tea tree oil added to the water. Or try one of these recipes:

Antifungal Salve

This salve was created for athlete's foot and works especially well for dry, chapped areas, lesions, and cracks. I have used this salve successfully for other fungal infections, as well as for mange on animals. If you can't find organically grown goldenseal, just omit it in this formula.

> 2 parts chaparral
> 2 parts black walnut hulls
> 1 part organically grown goldenseal
> 1 part myrrh
> 1 part echinacea
> a few drops of cajeput oil or tree tea oil

Follow instructions for making a salve on page 17. Apply twice daily, in the morning and evening. ❧

Antifungal Powder

This is an effective powder that is also simple to make. Use only organically grown goldenseal; if you can't find it, eliminate that ingredient from the recipe.

> ½ cup white cosmetic-grade clay or arrowroot powder
> 1 tablespoon chaparral powder
> 1 tablespoon black walnut hulls
> 1 teaspoon organically grown goldenseal
> 1 teaspoon tea tree oil

Mix clay or arrowroot powder, chaparral powder, black walnut hulls, and goldenseal. Add essential oil of tea tree and mix well. Let dry; store in a shaker bottle. Apply to feet once or twice daily.

Burns

Burns are damaged tissue caused by too much heat from fire, sun, or chemicals. First- and second-degree burns can generally be treated effectively at home, but you must be certain to keep the area clean to avoid infection. If infection should occur, seek medical advice. Always seek medical attention for third-degree burns.

What to Do

To treat a burn, first cool the area, thus "putting out the fire." Immerse the area in ice water or apply a diluted apple cider vinegar compress to the damaged area for at least a half hour. Next, choose one or more of the following treatments:

- Two to three drops of peppermint oil added to ¼ cup of honey makes a cooling disinfectant poultice for burns
- Aloe vera gel is cooling, disinfectant, and healing
- Valerian tincture taken internally helps alleviate pain
- For burns on the roof of the mouth from hot foods, make a pill ball (see recipe on page 20) with slippery elm and honey to heal the burn and lessen the pain

St.-John's-Wort Salve

St.-John's-wort salve or oil applied topically is especially helpful for healing burns and for any damaged nerve endings. This is an excellent, all-purpose salve also used for rashes, cuts, and wounds. I first made this salve back in 1974 and found it so effective I have been making it ever since.

1 part St.-John's-wort (leaves and flowers)
1 part comfrey leaf
1 part calendula flowers

Follow the instructions on page 17 for making a salve. Apply to the affected area 2–3 times daily.

Colds and Flus

Colds and flus are viral infections of the upper respiratory tract, often involving the throat, eyes, nose, and head. Bed rest is always recommended to treat these illnesses, but not always feasible. There are many other readily available, inexpensive treatments.

What to Do

Eat lightly, avoiding all dairy products and anything else that will cause more mucus in the system, such as sugar — including orange juice. Foods should be simple and warming. Hot broth was made for colds; drink it throughout the day. Add medicinal herbs such as astragalus and echinacea to the soup. And, of course, eat onions and garlic, nature's best remedies for colds and flus. Traditional curry blends are a mix of medicinal herbs, including turmeric and cayenne, which stimulate and activate the immune system. Sauté onion slices and whole cloves of garlic with lots of curry. It tastes divine, and clears the sinuses while effectively fighting the cold or flu virus.

Drink several cups a day of yarrow, peppermint, and elder tea (an old Gypsy formula) or hot ginger tea made from fresh grated ginger with honey and lemon. For an extra punch, I'll often sprinkle a bit of cayenne in the ginger tea. Both of these remedies will help you sweat out the cold.

Make your own echinacea tincture (see page 19 for instructions) before the cold season starts. In order for echinacea to ward off a cold, you must take ½ teaspoon of it every half hour at the first sign of infection. If you already have a cold, take 1 teaspoon of the tincture every two hours.

Fire Cider

This is another of my favorite remedies that is effective, easy to make, and tasty, but not for the weak at heart. Make a batch before the cold season starts.

> 1 quart vinegar
> ¼ cup grated fresh horseradish
> 1 chopped onion
> 1 head of garlic, peeled and chopped
> 2 tablespoons powdered turmeric
> cayenne
> 1 cup honey (more or less to taste)

1. Combine vinegar, horseradish, onion, garlic, turmeric, and a pinch or two of cayenne. Cover and let sit in a warm place for 3–4 weeks.
2. Strain mixture, add honey, and rebottle. Refrigerate. Take 1–2 tablespoons at the first sign of a cold and continue throughout the day (approximately every 2–3 hours) until the symptoms subside.

Conjunctivitis

A highly contagious inflammation of the eye, conjunctivitis causes the eyes to get red, swollen, and itchy. The tendency is to rub the itchy eye and then, unthinkingly, rub the other eye. Children often pass conjunctivitis among themselves.

What to Do

The immune system is often compromised when one contracts conjunctivitis; use echinacea to boost natural immunity. Administer ½ to 1 teaspoon every hour, decreasing the dosage as symptoms subside.

For severe itching, pain, and irritation, make a tea of equal amounts of lemon balm, lavender, and chamomile; drink several cups a day. Augment the relaxing and pain-relieving properties of the tea with one teaspoon of valerian tincture several times daily.

Eyewash

Use this eyewash to treat conjuntivitis without antibiotics. Be sure to strain the liquid well; you don't want any herb particles to get into the water. If you prefer, mix the herbs into a paste with a small amount of warm water, then spread the paste on a piece of gauze and apply as a poultice over the eyes.

> 1 teaspoon organically grown goldenseal root powder
> 1 tablespoon comfrey root powder
> 1 cup boiling water

1. Combine herbs and water. Strain well through two or three layers of muslin or a fine coffee filter. Allow liquid to cool to room temperature.
2. Using an eyecup or eye dropper, wash the eyes several times a day with the eyewash. Continue to apply daily until symptoms subside, usually within 4–5 days.

Constipation

Infrequent or difficult bowel movements are best treated with herbs. I would not recommend allopathic medicine for constipation; it is not designed to correct the situation, only remedy the symptoms. If constipation is chronic, consult a holistic health care practitioner.

What to Do

If you don't have a regular bowel movement at least once a day, consider constipation as a problem. When constipated, eliminate dietary factors that may be contributing to the problem; cheese, pasta, and bread are just a few of the foods that frequently cause constipation in people with sluggish bowels. For many people, stress and tension are the major causes of constipation; exercise is always helpful for eliminating constipation. Drink six to eight cups of pure water daily if constipation is a problem; constipation is often a result of insufficient hydration.

A good daily remedy is a mixture of one tablespoon each of ground psyllium seeds and ground flaxseed. Add the ground seeds to cereal, salads, or other foods. You must drink several cups of water daily when using these seeds.

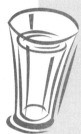

Yellow Dock Constipation Remedy

I've found yellow dock root to be excellent for constipation without any of the dependency issues. A tincture made from this formula may be used for difficult cases.

> 2 parts yellow dock root
> 1 part dandelion root
> 1 part licorice root

Make a decoction as instructed on page 14. Drink 3 cups daily.

Emergency Constipation Remedy

On occasion, when you need a good formula to get things going, try this one. Don't use it regularly, though, as the stronger herbs, senna and cascara, can create dependencies when used too often or too strongly.

> 1 part cascara sagrada
> 2 parts yellow dock root
> 3 parts licorice root
> 1 part senna
> 4 parts fennel seeds
> 1 part psyllium seeds

Mix herbs and make a decoction as directed on page 14. Drink 1–2 cups to start, and increase dose if needed.

Cuts, Wounds, and Bites

Lesions, open wounds, and surface cuts are often, though not always, accompanied by bleeding and pain. Large or deep wounds will need medical attention, but you can treat minor cuts at home.

What to Do

Wash any cuts out with an antiseptic solution consisting of witch hazel and tea tree oil (use 6 to 8 drops tea tree oil to 1 cup witch hazel extract). If necessary disinfect the area with Kloss's liniment (see recipe below).

To stop bleeding, apply a poultice or compress of shepherd's purse and yarrow. Apply topically until the wound stops bleeding. Believe it or not, clean cobwebs also will stop bleeding!

If the wound contains a splinter, soak in water and epsom salts, or apply a thick clay pack (green or red) directly to the spot. Leave it on for several hours; change once or twice during the day. Then disinfect the area with Kloss's liniment, lavender, or a similar remedy.

When the wound has been properly cleaned and the area disinfected, apply St.-John's-wort salve (see recipe on page 64). Wrap in a gauze bandage or cotton flannel cloth to keep clean and protected. If the cut is painful, drink lemon balm, valerian, and chamomile tea or tincture.

Kloss's Liniment

This liniment by that famous old herb doctor, Dr. Jethro Kloss, is useful for inflammation of the muscles, though I use it primarily as a disinfectant. If organically grown goldenseal isn't available, substitute chaparral or Oregon grape root.

- 1 ounce organically grown goldenseal powder
- 1 ounce echinacea powder
- 1 ounce myrrh powder
- ¼ ounce cayenne powder
- 1 pint rubbing alcohol

Follow the directions for making a tincture on page 19. Label clearly FOR EXTERNAL USE ONLY.

Goldenseal Salve

This salve is excellent when an astringent, disinfectant action is needed. It also serves as an emollient. If organically grown goldenseal is not available, substitute chaparral.

>   1 part organically grown goldenseal
>   1 part myrrh gum

Follow the instructions on page 17 for making salve. ⚘

Insect Repellent Oil

This insect repellent is quite safe for human and animal use.

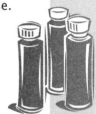

>   1 part fresh bay leaves
>   1 part eucalyptus leaves
>   2 parts rosemary
>   4 parts pennyroyal
>   cedarwood or eucalyptus essential oil

Use dried herbs or fresh wilt the leaves by allowing them to sit in a warm, shaded area for several hours, or until most of the water has evaporated. Follow the instructions on page 16 for making an herbal oil. Strain. Add a drop or two of essential oil to strengthen the scent. ⚘

Diarrhea

One of the most common ailments, diarrhea is characterized by loose, watery bowel movements. This problem can be caused by factors such as infection, unbalanced diet, and even stress. While everyone experiences diarrhea from time to time, if you have chronic diarrhea, you should consult a holistic health care practitioner or physician.

What to Do

Blackberry root tincture is my favorite remedy for diarrhea. At the first signs of diarrhea, take ½ teaspoon of tincture every half hour until symptoms subside. You may have to make your own, because it's seldom found in the herb shops; follow the directions for making tinctures on page 19.

If blackberry root is not available, any strong astringent such as white oak bark, witch hazel bark (not the extract sold in pharmacies), or raspberry leaf will do. Black tea also works in a pinch.

Use a tincture of mucilaginous herbs such as marsh mallow, licorice, and slippery elm to soothe the irritated bowels. Make a tea using two parts blackberry root and one part licorice root to augment the tincture. Drink three to four cups daily. If the diarrhea is persistent, add chaparral or cultivated goldenseal to the tea. Mix slippery elm with oatmeal porridge for a soothing, nonirritating, edible remedy.

It is essential to drink sufficient quantities of water when experiencing diarrhea; it is very easy to become dehydrated and ill as a result. Be especially mindful of this with small children, and ensure that their liquid intake is sufficient (several cups of water a day in addition to their medicinal tea).

Earache

Earaches are infections of the inner or outer ear signified by pain, redness, and sometimes itchiness around the outer ear. If the pain gets severe or is prolonged, consult a holistic health care provider or physician.

What to Do

Hot onion packs are an old-fashioned remedy that really works. Wrap hot sautéed onions in a flannel cloth and apply directly to both ears (one at a time, if desired). Reheat the onions as needed. Leave the hot onion pack on for 30–45 minutes, longer if possible.

If the onion pack doesn't work, heat some salt in a cast-iron skillet; when it is too hot to touch, pour it onto a dish-cloth or cotton cloth. Fold carefully, being sure not to burn yourself. Using other towels to protect against the heat, place against the ear for at least 30 minutes. Treat both ears.

Generally, earaches are accompanied by colds and flus. Treat the related symptoms, and eliminate foods that may be congesting to the eardrums. Dairy, sugar, and citrus products (with the exception of lemons and grapefruit) are the primary

TREATING SWIMMER'S EAR

Swimmer's ear is an ear infection that is caused by water in the eardrum. It doesn't respond well to oil applications. Instead, combine several drops of tea tree or lavender oil with ¼ cup of rubbing alcohol. Shake well. Using a dropper, apply several drops in each ear. Massage the outer ear. Repeat several times daily, until symptoms subside. Hot salt packs (see page 70) are often helpful for swimmer's ear.

culprits. Take ½ to 1 teaspoon of echinacea tincture several times a day to activate the immune system.

Garlic-Mullein Flower Oil

This is a wonderful remedy for ear infections that relieves the pain and helps eliminate the infection. St.-John's-wort oil is often added to this blend to enhance its effectiveness. The flowers of mullein are often difficult to purchase, so gather some in the summer and fall.

> 2–3 tablespoons chopped garlic
> 2–3 tablespoons mullein flowers
> virgin olive oil

Follow the directions on page 16 for making an herbal oil. Warm only to body temperature and apply 3–4 drops into each ear. Massage the outer ear and around the base of the ear after applying the oil. Repeat several times daily.

Fevers

Any temperature over 98.6°F, the perfect human body temperature, is considered a fever. Fever is the immune system's natural defense for stopping infection and disease. However, out-of-control fevers can be devastating. A fever over 104°F should receive immediate attention by a holistic health care provider; if the sick person is a child, though, do not wait for the fever to climb this high.

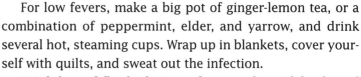

What to Do

For low fevers, make a big pot of ginger-lemon tea, or a combination of peppermint, elder, and yarrow, and drink several hot, steaming cups. Wrap up in blankets, cover yourself with quilts, and sweat out the infection.

Drink lots of fluids during a fever, and avoid foods and drinks that are dehydrating (coffee, black tea, soda water). Use ½ to 1 teaspoon echinacea tincture several times daily to boost the immune system. Wrap the forehead and feet with washcloths dipped in cold water with a few drops of lavender oil added to it.

Catnip enemas are one of the very best techniques for lowering a fever and hydrating the system, especially in children. You will need an appropriate size enema bag with a pressure regulator on the tubing. Be sure to use an infant or child's size enema bag for the little ones. Consult your healthcare provider before administering enemas, and only use them in extreme cases when liquids are not tolerated.

Cold Wraps

Cold sheet wraps are one of the best techniques for lowering fever, hydrating the system, and improving circulation. Fine salons often combine cold wraps with aromatherapy as a high-priced beauty treatment.

Cold wraps are administered in bed, which will need to be protected with plastic sheeting. Soak a bedsheet in a large pan of cold or tepid water. Essential oils such as lavender, eucalyptus, tea tree, cajeput, pine, or cedar added to the water or sprinkled on the sheet enhance the therapeutic value of these wraps. Wring the sheet completely, then place it on the plastic sheeting. Instruct the person to lay down in the middle of the sheet and wrap it snugly around him, from toes to neck — leave only the head protruding. Place a tepid damp cloth on the forehead.

This treatment should be administered for 15 to 20 minutes only. Do not let the person get chilled; be sure the temperature of the room is warm. After the wrap, serve a large cup of warm ginger tea, and put the person directly into a warm, comfy bed.

Heartburn

This unpleasant burning sensation behind the breastbone — sometimes accompanied by a sulfurlike flavor in the mouth — is caused by spasms and irritation in the esophagus or upper stomach. Heartburn is a sure sign that you are offending your stomach in some manner. Stress, too much food, and a too-rich diet are common causes of heartburn.

What to Do

The best herbs to use for heartburn are plants that calm the nervous system and are good digestive nervines, such as chamomile, hops, and lemon balm. Mucilaginous herbs will soothe the irritated stomach lining.

Drink an infusion of 1 part licorice, 1 part chamomile, and 2 parts lemon balm a half hour before and after meals to prevent heartburn. Use a digestive bitter such as Swedish Bitters (available in herb and natural foods stores) and/or hops tincture with every meal.

Peppermint tea is often a very helpful preventive; drink before and after meals. Try adding a drop or two of peppermint essential oil to water and drinking small sips during the meal.

Relax during and after meals. Try deep breathing, offering prayer before your meal, and chewing slowly, counting your chews. Don't eat when you're upset; take a walk instead.

Headaches

Headaches, typified by throbbing or dull pain in the head, have a variety of causes, ranging from eating too much too fast to emotional factors. They are a sure sign that things are "not OK," at least for the moment.

What to Do

Most headaches respond well to simple care. Try any or all of these treatments:

Lavender oil bath. Baths are soothing, and lavender oil enhances the calming effect. If a full bath is not possible, use lavender oil in a hot herbal foot bath. Rubbing the shoulders while the feet are soaking is often helpful in kissing that headache good-bye. You may also wrap the head in a cool cloth sprinkled with lavender oil.

Valerian tincture. Used for stress-related headaches, valerian tincture is extremely effective. Take ¼ teaspoon of the tincture every half hour until symptoms subside.

Salted plums and miso soup. If the headache is of the vascular type caused by a rich diet, too much sugar, or a highly charged emotional state rather than stress factors, try eating Japanese salted plums or a cup of miso soup. This will alkalize the blood quickly, changing the pH, and often will diminish the headache.

Headache Tea

Different people respond to different headache remedies. This is one of my favorite combinations; it also makes a great tincture for headaches and migraines alike. Headache Tea is even more effective if used in conjunction with a hot lavender oil bath.

> 1 part feverfew
> 2 parts lemon balm
> 1 part lavender

Make a tea following the directions on page 12. Drink ¼ cup every half hour. ⁓

Treating Migraines

Migraines are a headache unto themselves: excruciatingly painful, recurring, and often difficult to treat. If you grow feverfew, eat a leaf or two daily. It can also be dried and used in tea; drink a cup or two daily. I recommend tincturing this herb with lavender; take one teaspoon daily as a preventive. Feverfew often works for people when nothing else has. It must be used over a period of at least three months before determining if it works, however. Feverfew is not recommended during pregnancy.

When you feel a migraine coming on, mix ½ teaspoon of guarana with two packages of Alacer's Emergen-C (a source of vitamin C found in natural foods stores). Repeat if necessary. If guarana is not available, take a large dose of coffee. It may keep you up, but often it averts the headache.

Indigestion and Poor Digestion

The inablity to digest foods creates sluggish elimination, gas, and poor assimilation of nutrients. Poor digestion and pain and gas in the abdomen are usually a result of poor eating habits, low-quality food, and stress. Therefore, indigestion responds well to lifestyle changes. Low digestive enymes and intestinal flora can also result in digestive problems.

What to Do

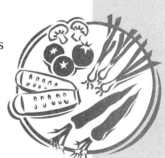

Before changing your diet or adding supplements and herbs, try these simple suggestions:

- Say a prayer before your meal; honor the food that you're about to eat.
- Chew slowly and thoughtfully. If engaging in conversation, keep voices quiet and conversation peaceful.
- Don't rush through your meal. Imagine this as your last one and enjoy it.
- Don't drink cold fluids with your meal; in fact, it's best not to drink immediately before or after a meal.
- Be careful of what foods you combine at meals. Carbohydrates and protein, combined in our American meal plans, ensure gas and putrefaction in the system. Educate yourself to proper food combinations that aid digestion.

In addition to changing your habits:

- Drink a peppermint and chamomile tea a half hour before and after meals.
- Buy a ready-made digestive bitter such as Swedish Bitters (available at health foods stores) or make your own digestive bitter tincture.

- Add ginger and cayenne to your food or make a warm tea with them if you have slow digestion. Use fresh grated ginger and only a few grains of cayenne.
- Take papaya enzymes with meals to aid digestion.
- Take a daily supplement of acidophilus. This product restores weak intestinal flora and is readily available at every natural foods store.
- Combine carminitive seeds and chew them at and between meals. Dill, cardamon, anise, fennel, and cumin, are all very helpful for reducing gas and bloated stomachs.

Digestive Bitter Tincture

1 part gentian
1 part artichoke leaf
2 parts fennel
1 part dandelion root
½ part ginger

Combine herbs and follow directions on page 19 for making a tincture. Take ½–1 teaspoon before and after meals. ❧

Insomnia

Sleeplessness or restless sleep is a big problem when it hits someone already anxious or stressed. The body needs to sleep in order to produce essential hormones and to dream. Our dreams are important to our health and psyche, whether we remember them or not.

What to Do

This program is my favorite solution for insomnia — it works almost every time. Take ½ teaspoon St.-John's-wort tincture three times daily for five days, stop for two days; then repeat the cycle until you're able to sleep peacefully.

Throughout the day, drink a good nervine tea such as a blend of lemon balm, chamomile, and passionflower, stopping three hours before bedtime — you don't want to wake up to

TIP FOR RESTFUL SLEEP

If you should wake up in the night, don't try to go back to sleep. Instead, sit up, turn your light on and begin to read the most boring book you can possibly find. It must be boring and unreadable, not a fascinating novel. Continue to take the hops-valerian tincture that you keep next to your bed. Have a good night's sleep.

use the bathroom! Or take one teaspoon of a combination hops and valerian tincture beginning two or three hours before bedtime, and continuing each hour until you go to bed.

Just before bed, take either a warm lavender oil bath or an invigorating walk outdoors. If you're walking on grass and it's possible to go barefoot, do so. It connects you to the electromagnetic forces of the Earth. Jump into bed following your bath or walk. Usually you'll go right to sleep.

Laryngitis or Sore Throat

Though sore throats and laryngitis are not technically the same, they respond to the same treatments. Laryngitis is inflammation of the throat, resulting in hoarseness and often, though not always, a sore throat. It is generally a result of an infection or stressed vocal cords. Sore throats are always a result of infection and don't necessarily result in laryngitis.

What to Do

The best and surest thing to do for laryngitis is to rest the voice. Several herbal companies make excellent throat sprays incorporating echinacea, licorice, slippery elm, and other herbs specific to irritated vocal cords. Make your own by brewing a triple-strength tea of licorice, echinacea, and sage (3 teaspoons of herb per cup) and add a few drops of tea tree or eucalyptus oil to it. Put the mix in a mister or spray bottle and squirt into the back of the throat as needed.

Garden sage is often used by people for sore throats and laryngitis. Use it as both a tea and a gargle.

Throat Soother Tea

This tea strengthens the voice and soothes throat irritation.

>   1 part marsh mallow root
>   2 parts licorice root
>   1 part echinacea
>   1 part cinnamon
>   ⅛ part ginger

Decoct herbs as instructed on page 14. Drink several cups of tea a day. ❧

Sore Throat Gargle

This is my favorite gargle for sore throats and laryngitis; however, I'm the first to admit that it's not my tastiest recipe.

>   1 cup strong sage tea (triple strength)
>   1 cup apple cider vinegar
> 2–3 cups salt
>   pinch of cayenne

Combine all ingredients. Gargle with this mixture frequently throughout the day. ❧

Cough Be Gone & Sore Throat Syrup

This syrup for sore and inflamed throats is a much tastier recipe than my Sore Throat Gargle.

>   2 parts slippery elm bark
>   2 parts valerian
>   2 parts wild cherry bark
>   2 parts licorice root
>   4 parts fennel seeds
>   1 part cinnamon bark
>   ½ part gingerroot
>   ⅛ part orange peel

Make a syrup as instructed on page 15. Take 1–2 teaspoons every hour or two throughout the day, or use whenever a bout of coughing starts up. ❧

Throat Balls

This tasty herbal candy is excellent for sore or strep throat. If organically grown goldenseal is unavailable, substitute Oregon grape root.

   1 part licorice root powder
   1 part carob powder
   1 part slippery elm or marsh mallow powder
   ½ part echinacea powder
   ¼ part organically grown goldenseal powder
   a few drops of peppermint oil

Make a batch of herbal candy as instructed on page 15. Add more carob to thicken, and adjust flavors to suit you. Take 1 marble-sized ball 3–4 times daily.

Poison Oak, Poison Ivy

A hot, itchy rash caused by beautiful woodland vines, poison oak is the culprit on the west coast, and poison ivy on the east. This contact dermatitis can get quite severe in sensitive people.

What to Do

I've used Kloss's liniment (page 68) successfully for stopping the itch and spread of poison oak and ivy. Dilute it with water or witch hazel extract so it stings but doesn't burn. Keep the bottle handy and apply frequently throughout the day.

In areas where it's not possible to use the liniment or a drying clay due to sensitivity (genitals and eyes), use unsweetened yogurt. This was my grandmother's favorite remedy when I had poison oak as a child. She would cover me with her tart Armenian yogurt and leave me to dry. It was uncomfortable, but it worked.

Assist the body in healing by taking echinacea tincture throughout the day. Since the rash produces a "hot" condition in the body, it is important to use cooling herbs to help with the symptoms. Cleavers, chickweed, burdock, and dandelion are all recommended. Make a tea with a combination of these herbs; drink several cups a day.

TIPS FOR COPING WITH POISON OAK AND POISON IVY

For the irritation, which at times can be unbearable, take large doses of kava-kava and/or valerian tincture. As a distraction, read a good novel or watch some spellbinding videos. If you tend to scratch the rash at night, which is common, do what parents to do infants: cover your hands with socks at night. When worse comes to worst, remember, this too shall pass. The affliction always runs its course.

Along similar lines, avoid spicy foods, as they will agitate the heat condition and make the itch worse. Though it's tempting to take a hot bath or shower, and it will make the rash feel better temporarily, it will always agitate the condition in the long run. Avoid hot baths, showers, saunas, and sweat lodges. Bathe only in tepid water.

Ocean water is one of the most healing treatments for these rashes. If you don't live near the sea and are unable to bathe in it daily, simulate the ocean waters in your tub: add kelp, baking soda, and sea salt to the tub, cool water only. A drop or two of peppermint oil (no more or you'll be flying out of that tub before you get in it!) will help cool the rash and give temporary relief from the burning.

Itch Relief Remedy

My favorite remedy for poison oak/ivy was a French-made toothpaste containing green clay, salt, water, and peppermint oil. The company has gone out of business, but the remedy is easy to make. Store this wonderful healing cream in a glass container with a tight-fitting lid. If it dries out, reconstitute by adding water.

> 1 cup green volcanic clay
> water or witch hazel extract
> 2 tablespoons salt
> peppermint oil

1. Mix the clay with enough water or witch hazel extract to make a creamy paste. Add salt and several drops of peppermint; the paste should smell strong and feel cooling to the skin.
2. Spread directly on affected area and leave on until it's completely dry. To rinse off, soak a washcloth in witch hazel extract or water and rub gently. Don't scrub the skin. ❧

Toothache

Who hasn't had one of these? A toothache can be caused by stress or anxiety, but is generally caused by bacteria infecting the tissue at the base of the tooth. The pain is the irritated nerve sending a signal that something is awry.

What to Do

Make an appointment to see a good dentist. In the meantime, you can alleviate and often cure a toothache by applying poultices of herbs directly to the site of infection (see recipe below). Clove oil applied topically is an effective analgesic for toothaches, helping to relieve the pain. Valerian, if taken in sufficiently high dosages (½ teaspoon of the tincture every half hour) will also help lessen the pain. Spilanthes, too, has antiseptic and analgesic properties. In addition, tea tree oil can be applied directly to the infection. For recurring toothaches, examine your diet, lifestyle, and dental hygiene habits.

Toothache Poultice

Substitute chaparral in this formula if organically grown goldenseal is not available.

    1 part organically grown goldenseal
    1 part myrrh
    1 part spilanthes (if available)
    1 part turmeric
    1 drop clove oil

Powder the herbs and mix into a thick paste with water. Add clove oil as an analgesic and antiseptic. Make a small cylinder-shaped poultice and apply directly to the affected area. ❧

Healing Mouthwash

This mouthwash has helped lessen my trips to the dentist.

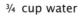

- ¾ cup water
- ¼ cup vodka
- 2 droppersful organically grown goldenseal or chaparral tincture
- 2 droppersful calendula tincture
- 1 dropperful myrrh tincture
- 1–2 drops essential oil of peppermint

Mix water and vodka. Add tinctures and shake well. Dilute several tablespoons of the mixture in ½ ounce of water, and use as a mouthwash.

Urinary Tract Infections and Cystitis

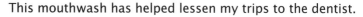

Cystitis is an infection of the bladder and urinary system. Symptoms include difficult, burning urination, feeling like one has to urinate but is unable to, low energy, and sometimes fever. This type of infection can be dangerous if involving the kidneys, so be mindful and treat it right away.

What to Do

Cystitis is generally easy to treat with home remedies. Begin treatment at the first signs of cystitis: slight burning when urinating or incomplete emptying of the bladder. If you follow even some of these suggestions, the cystitis should be cleared up in a day or two. If it persists for longer than seven days, consult a holistic health care practitioner.

Bed rest is always recommended. Your body is trying to fight off an infection, so slow down.

Take herbs used specifically for cystitis, such as uva ursi, pipsissewa, buchu, cleavers, chickweed, nettle, and dandelion leaf. Combine two or more of these to make a tea; drink several cups a day. Take several teaspoons of echinacea tincture daily to boost your resistance.

Cranberry juice prevents bacteria from adhering to the kidneys and urethra and is one of the best preventives and remedies for urinary tract infections. Drink several cups a day.

Though unsweetened cranberry juice is best (it is very tart, so you may wish to dilute it with tea or apple juice), Ocean Spray does work.

Drink adequate amounts of water when you're suffering from cystitis. Fill a quart bottle with water and add the juice of one or two lemons and a squirt of uva ursi tincture.

Keep the kidney area warm. Don't expose the kidney area to cold water or cold air. Place a hot-water bottle over the kidneys at night and whenever you're sitting. If you must go to work, take your hot-water bottle with you. Wear long sweaters that cover the kidney area.

Do not make love when you have a urinary infection. It is not contagious, but lovemaking can irritate the condition.

Eat lots of yogurt and miso or chicken soup. Alcohol and sugary foods will agitate cystitis. Drink warm teas to soothe the pain and boost the body's natural defenses.

Cystitis Remedy

This is an excellent infection-fighting formula for cystitis.

2 parts uva ursi
2 parts fresh or dried cranberries
1 part chickweed
2 parts cleavers
1 part marsh mallow root

Brew as an infusion, following the directions on page 13. Drink 4 cups daily, ¼ cup a time. 🪰

Warts

Warts are viral infections that appear as hard, knotty little protrusions on the skin. Although they are unsightly and annoying, they rarely cause serious problems.

What to Do

Warts are among the most mysterious of all things to treat. They can respond to a plethora of different approaches — from throwing a beefsteak over your left shoulder to burning them off with chemicals. Sometimes they respond to nothing at all. Over the years I've heard of a variety of different treatments that have worked for people. Here's a list of some of the most effective treatments:

- The inside of a ripe banana peel applied topically is the recommended remedy of Cascade Anderson Geller and David Winston, both renowned herbalists. Tape the inner peel of the banana over the wart; change several times daily. It may take two or three weeks of this treatment, but they swear it works.
- A poultice of raw eggplant applied topically has been reported by several people as having excellent results. Change once a day. Again, this treatment may take two or three weeks.
- Antiviral essential oils such as tea tree, cajeput, and thuja have been applied topically for several weeks with some success.
- Kloss's liniment and cayenne packs directly on warts have been successful for me.
- A tincture made with equal parts black walnut, echinacea, and pau d'arco is effective if warts are of the spreading type; take ½ teaspoon three times a day, and apply topically, as well
- You can try my method of getting rid of warts. When I was 13, I was awkward, thin, with long dark hair. You can imagine my chagrin when a wart appeared on my chin. I looked at it every day in the mirror, stared it down, and told it to go away. In seven days it was gone.

Resources

Where to Find Herbs

Thankfully, herbs and herbal products are now widely available. I generally suggest purchasing herbal products from local sources, as it helps support bioregional herbalism and community-based herbalists. However, here are some of my favorite sources for high-quaility herbs and herbal products.

Frontier Herbs
P.O. Box 299
Norway, IA 52318
(800) 669-3275
Aside from having an incredible list of supplies and herbs, Frontier emphasizes medicinal plant conservation and preservation. Frontier is a wholesale supplier, but offers price breaks for individual buyers.

Green Mountain Herbs
P.O. Box 532
Putney, VT 05436
(888) 4GRNMTS

Healing Spirits
9198 State Route 415
Avoca, NY 14809
(607) 566-2701
One of the best sources of ethically wildcrafted and organically grown herbs in the northeast.

Jean's Greens
119 Sulphur Springs Road
Newport, NY 13146
(315) 845-6500
A wonderful selection of fresh and dried organic and wildcrafted herbs. Also, oils, containers, beeswax, and other materials needed for making herbal products.

Mountain Rose
20818 High Street
North San Juan, CA 95960
(800) 879-3337
A small herb company nestled in the coastal mountains of northern California, that supplies bulk herbs, beeswax, books, oils, and containers.

Trinity Herbs
P.O. Box 1001
Graton, CA 95444
(707) 824-2040
Trinity is a small wholesale herb company that sells bulk herbs in quantities of one pound or more.

Wild Weeds
1302 Camp Weott Road
Ferndale, CA 95536
(800) 553-9453
A small herbal emporium, this mail-order business was initially started to supply correspondence-course students with the herbs and herbal materials they needed.

Woodland Essences
P.O. Box 206
Cold Brook, NY 13324
(315) 845-1515

Handmade Herbal Products

Each of the following companies provides high-quality herbal products. Write for their current catalogs and price lists.

Avena Botanicals
20 Mill Street
Rockland, ME 04841

Equinox Botanicals
33446 McCumber Road
Rutland, OH 45775

Green Terrestrial
P.O. Box 266
Milton, NY 12547

Herb Pharm
Box 116
Williams, OR 97544

Herbalists and Alchemists
P.O. Box 553
Broadway, NJ 08808

Sage Mountain Herb Products
General Delivery
Lake Elmore, VT 05657
(802) 888-7278
Rosemary Gladstar's company.

Simpler's Botanicals
P.O. Box 39
Forestville, CA 95436

Zand Herbal Products
Products available in most natural foods and herb stores.

Educational Resources

A few years ago it was difficult to find herbal educational opportunities, but today the choices are many. Following are a few well-known herbal schools and programs.

American Herb Association (AHA)
P.O. Box 1673
Nevada City, CA 95959
More complete listings of schools, programs, seminars, and correspondence courses offered throughout the United States. There is a small fee for this publication.

American Herbalist Guild (AHG)
Box 746555
Arvada, CO 80006
More complete listings of schools, programs, seminars, and correspondence courses offered throughout the United States. There is a small fee for this publication.

The California School of Herbal Studies
P.O. Box 39
Forestville, CA 95476
One of the oldest and most respected herb schools in the United States, founded by Rosemary Gladstar in 1982.

Herb Research Foundation
1007 Pearl Street, Suite 200
Boulder, CO 80302
An excellent resource and research organization. They also have a newsletter.

**The Northeast Herb
Association**
P.O. Box 10
Newport, NY 13416

**Rocky Mountain Center for
Botanical Studies**
1705 Fourteenth Street, #287
Boulder, CO 80302
*Offers excellent programs
for beginners, as well as
advanced clinical training
programs.*

**Sage Mountain Retreat
Center and Botanical
Sanctuary**
P.O. Box 420
East Barre, VT 05649
*Apprentice programs and
classes with Rosemary
Gladstar and other well-
known herbalists.*

**The Science and Art
of Herbalism: A Home
Study Course**
by Rosemary Gladstar
P.O. Box 420
East Barre, VT 05649
*The Science and Art of Herbal-
ism was written in an inspir-
ing and joyful manner for
students wishing a systematic,
in-depth study of herbs. The
course emphasizes the foun-
dations of herbalism, wildcrafting, Earth awareness,
and herbal preparation and
formulation. The heart of the
course is the development of a
deep personal relationship
with the plant world.*

Herb Newsletters

*The American Herb
Association Newsletter*
P.O. Box 1673
Nevada City, CA 95959

Business of Herbs
North Winds Farm
439 Pondersona Way
Jemez Springs, NM 87025

*Foster's Botanical and
Herb Reviews*
P.O. Box 106
Eureka Springs, AR 72632

HerbalGram
P.O. Box 201660
Austin, TX 78720

The Herb Quarterly
P.O. Box 548
Boiling Springs, PA 17007

Herbs for Health and *The
Herb Companion*
201 East Fourth Street
Loveland, CO 80537

Medical Herbalism
P.O. Box 33080
Portland, OR 97233

*Planetary Formula
Newsletter*
c/o Roy Upton
P.O. Box 533
Soquel, CA 95073

United Plant Savers
P.O. Box 420
East Barre, VT 05649

Wild Foods Forum
4 Carlisle Way NE
Atlanta, GA 30308

United Plant Savers At-Risk List

United Plant Savers (UpS) is a nonprofit, grassroots organization dedicated to preserving native American medicinal plants and the land that they grow on. An organization for herbalists and people who love and use plants, our purpose is to ensure the future of our rich diversity of medicinal plants through organic cultivation, sustainable wildcrafting practices, creating botanical sanctuaries for medicinal plant conservation, and reestablishing native plant communities in their natural environments.

The following herbs have been designated as "UpS At Risk" due to overharvesting, loss of habitat, or by nature of their innate rareness or sensitivity. UpS is not asking for a moratorium on the use of these herbs, but rather is asking for a concerted effort by all those who use plants as medicine to seek sustainable alternatives; that is, grow your own, buy from reputable companies, or substitute other herbs whenever possible.

American Ginseng *(Panax quinquefolius)*

Black Cohosh *(Cimicifuga racemosa)*

Bloodroot *(Sanguinaria canadensis)*

Blue Cohosh *(Caulophyllum thalictroides)*

Echinacea (*Echinacea* species)

Goldenseal *(Hydrastis canadensis)*

Helonias Root *(Chamaelirium luteum)*

Kava-Kava *(Piper methysticum)* (Hawaii only)

Lady's-Slipper (*Cypripedium* species)

Lomatium *(Lomatium dissectum)*

Osha (*Ligusticum porteri* and related species)

Partridgeberry *(Mitchella repens)*

Peyote *(Lophophora williamsii)*

Slippery elm *(Ulmus rubra)*

Sundew (*Drosera* species)

Trillium, Beth root (*Trillium* species)

True Unicorn *(Aletris farinosa)*

Venus's-flytrap *(Dionaea muscipula)*

Wild Yam *(Dioscorea villosa* and related species)

For more information on United Plant Savers and how you can become involved in "Planting the Future," contact United Plant Savers, P.O. Box 98, East Barre, VT 05649; (802) 479-9825; E-mail: info@www.plantsavers.org.

Index

Sage *(Salvia officinalis)*, 45, 60, 77, 78
Salt packs, 70
Salves, 17–18, 62, 64, 69
Saw palmetto *(Serenoa repens)*, 46
Senna, 67
Shepherd's purse, 68
Slippery elm *(Ulmus fulva)*, 47, 63, 70, 77, 78, 79
Sore throat, 77–79
Spearmint *(Mentha spicata)*, 47
Spilanthes, 81
Splinters, 68
St.-John's-wort *(Hypericum perforatum)*, 45–46, 64, 68, 71, 76
Stevia *(Stevia rebundiana)*, 48
Storing herbs, 9–10
Swedish Bitters, 73, 75
Swimmer's ear, 71
Syrups, herbal, 15, 78

Teas, herbal, 11–14. *See also specific teas, herbs, or illnesses*
Tea tree, 63, 68, 77, 81, 83
Throat Balls, 79
Throat Soother Tea, 78
Thyme, 60
Tinctures, 18–20, 76
Tools, for making herbal products, 10

Toothache, 81–82
Toxicity, of herbs, 5–6
Turmeric, 60, 65

United Plant Savers at-risk list, 89
Urinary track infections, 82–83
Usnea *(Usnea barbata)*, 48
Uva ursi *(Arctostaphylos uva-ursi)*, 49, 82, 83

Valerian *(Valeriana officinalis)*, 49, 63, 66, 68, 74, 77, 78, 80, 81

Warts, 83–84
White oak *(Quercus alba)*, 50, 70
Wild cherry *(Prunus serotina)*, 50, 78
Wild yam *(Dioscorea villosa)*, 51
Witch hazel *(Hamamelis virginiana)*, 51, 68, 70, 80
Wounds, 68–69

Yarrow *(Achillea millefolium)*, 52, 64, 68, 72
Yellow dock *(Rumex crispus)*, 52, 67
Yogurt, 79

Other Storey Books You Will Enjoy

Also in the Rosemary Gladstar Series: *Remedies for Children's Health,* ISBN 1-58017-153-2; *Herbal Remedies for Men's Health,* ISBN 1-58017-151-6; *Herbs for Longevity and Well-Being,* ISBN 1-58017-154-0; *Herbs for Natural Beauty,* ISBN 1-58017-152-4; and *Herbs for Reducing Stress and Anxiety,* ISBN 1-58017-155-9.

Healing with Herbs, by Penelope Ody. This visual introduction to the world of herbal medicine offers clear, illustrated instructions for growing, preparing, and administering healing herbs to relieve a variety of ailments. 160 pages. Hardcover. ISBN 1-58017-144-3.

Herbal Antibiotics, by Stephen Harrod Buhner. This book presents all the current information about antibiotic-resistant microbes and the herbs that are most effective in fighting them. Readers will also find detailed, step-by-step instructions for making and using herbal infusions, tinctures, teas, and salves to treat various types of infections. 128 pages. Paperback. ISBN 1-58017-148-6.

The Herbal Home Remedy Book, by Joyce A. Wardwell. Discover how to use 25 common herbs to make simple herbal remedies. Native American legends and folklore are spread throughout the book. 176 pages. Paperback. ISBN 1-58017-016-1.

Herbal Remedy Gardens, by Dorie Byers. An introduction to more than 20 herbs, their medicinal uses, propagation, and harvesting techniques, this book includes dozens of easy-to-make recipes for common ailments. Thirty-eight illustrated garden plans offer choices for customizing a garden to fit your special health needs. 224 pages. Paperback. ISBN 1-58017-095-1.

Herbal Tea Gardens, by Marietta Marshall Marcin. This tea lover's gardening bible contains full instructions for growing and brewing tea herbs, plus more than 100 recipes that make use of their healthful qualities. Complete plans for customized gardens suitable for plots or containers. 192 pages. ISBN 1-58017-106-0.

Natural First Aid, by Brigitte Mars. This book offers natural first-aid suggestions for everything from ant bites to wounds. Readers will also find recipes for simple home remedies using herbs, vitamins, essential oils, and foods. Includes an herb profile section detailing the healing properties of common herbs. 128 pages. Paperback. ISBN 1-58017-147-8.

These and other Storey books are available at your bookstore, farm store, garden center, or directly from Storey Books, Schoolhouse Road, Pownal, Vermont 05261, or by calling 1-800-441-5700. Or visit our Web site at www.storey.com.